ORYX SCIENCE BIBLIOGRAPHIES

Volume 8

Alzheimer's Disease

Compiled by Margaret Eide and
Twyla Mueller Racz
David A. Tyckoson, Series Editor

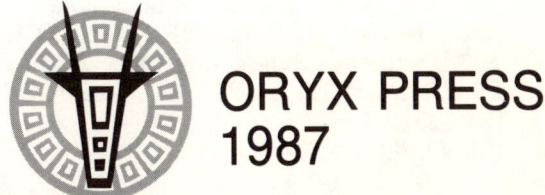

ORYX PRESS
1987

The rare Arabian Oryx is believed to have inspired the myth of the unicorn. This desert antelope became virtually extinct in the early 1960s. At that time several groups of international conservationists arranged to have 9 animals sent to the Phoenix Zoo to be the nucleus of a captive breeding herd. Today the Oryx population is over 400, and herds have been returned to reserves in Israel, Jordan, and Oman.

Copyright © 1987 by David A. Tyckoson

Published by The Oryx Press
2214 North Central at Encanto
Phoenix, AZ 85004-1483

Published simultaneously in Canada

All rights reserved
No part of this publication may be reproduced or transmitted in any form or by any means, electronic or mechanical, including photocopying, recording, or by any information storage and retrieval system, without permission in writing from The Oryx Press.

Printed and Bound in the United States of America

Library of Congress Cataloging-in-Publication Data

Eide, Margaret.
   Alzheimer's Disease.

  (Oryx science bibliographies ; v. 8)
  Includes index.
  1. Alzheimer's disease—Bibliography. I. Mueller Racz, Twyla. II. Title. III. Series. [DNLM:
1. Alzheimer's Disease—abstracts. ZWM 220 E34a]
Z6665.7.A45E37   1987   016.61897′683   86-28609
[RC523]
ISBN 0-89774-324-5

Table of Contents

About the Series	1
Research Review: Alzheimer's Disease	3
Alzheimer's Disease	9
Symptoms and Causes of Alzheimer's Disease	20
Diagnosis	25
Care and Treatment	29
Research on Alzheimer's Disease	38
Case Studies, Clinical Reports, and Statistics	50
Personal Narratives	54
Psychological and Social Aspects of Alzheimer's Disease	59
Author Index	68

About the Series

The <u>Oryx Science Bibliographies</u> are a new series of bibliographies designed to bring you the most recent references on the current issues in the sciences. Each issue will provide between 200-300 fully annotated references along with a "Research Review" covering the history and state of the art of the topic being covered. These bibliographies are intended to provide the student or researcher with an effective introduction to the hot topics in the sciences. Each bibliography also contains a number of special features, such as:

Evaluative Selection: The bibliographer reviews each article to ensure that only the most valuable references are included. The bibliography does not strive to be comprehensive but to include only the most important items on the topic.

Fully Annotated: All of the references are annotated, providing a useful summary of the source material for the user.

Readily Available Materials: All references chosen for inclusion are available at most libraries throughout the United States and Canada. Obscure sources that are difficult to obtain are usually avoided.

Highly Current: The bibliography strives to include the most recent materials to keep it as up to date as possible. References from as recently as the last six months before publication may be found in all issues.

Key Articles Highlighted: The most important articles in each bibliography are highlighted in **boldface** so that the user interested in only a few materials can key in to those that are the most useful.

Research Review: Each issue contains a research review describing the state of the art of the subject being covered.

Undergraduate Level: Only materials that are written at the undergraduate student level are chosen. Neither highly technical nor extremely general articles are included.

English Language Only: Only English language materials are included.

Research Review: Alzheimer's Disease

Two incurable diseases that affect special populations have recieved extensive news coverage during the 1980s. One is a newly discovered syndrome that has killed tens of thousands of victims; the other has been known throughout this century and involves millions of patients. Both lead to the total incapacitation and eventual death of the victim. Neither disease can be directly identified and neither has a known cure or treatment. The first of the two is AIDS, which has been the subject of two previous bibliographies in this series. The second is Alzheimer's disease, which is much more widespread and equally as deadly.

Alzheimer's Disease

Alzheimer's disease was first identified and described in November 1906 by the German physician Alois Alzheimer. He had observed a female patient with symptoms of memory loss, disorientation, depression, hallucinations, and eventually severe dementia and death. An autopsy of the patient's brain showed severe atrophy of the cerebral cortex and a clumping and distortion of fibers in the nerve cells of the brain. These neurofibrillary tangles have become the unique identifying factor of Alzheimer's disease. This disease has since been distinguished from the normal aging process and has technically become known as Senile Dementia of the Alzheimer Type (SDAT). With the increased lifespan brought about by modern society, Alzheimer's disease is becoming an increasingly important and deadly syndrome.

Symptoms

The onset of Alzheimer's disease is a slow and almost imperceptible process. At first, the victim experiences only minor memory lapses that are often attributed to emotional upsets or physical illnesses. Gradually the person becomes more and more forgetful, especially in relation to recent events. Eventually memory loss becomes highly significant and other changes, such as confusion, irritability, restlessness, and agitation are likely to appear in the victim's personality, mood, and behavior. Judgement, concentration, and speech may also be affected and, in the most severe cases, the victim is totally incapable of self-care. While these symptoms are progressive, there is a wide variety in the rate of change from person to person. The victim is often unaware of the disease or will not admit the severity of the condition. Alzheimer's disease significantly reduces the lifespan of many of its victims.

Diagnosis

The only definitive diagnosis for Alzheimer's disease is through an autopsy of the victim's brain to identify the specific neurofibrillary tangles associated with the disease. Since this can only be done after the death of the patient, physicians must make a living diagnosis of Alzheimer's disease by excluding any other possible causes of the symptoms observed. Many treatable psychiatric disorders, such as severe depression, are often misdiagnosed as Alzheimer's. It is important to eliminate any of these possibilities before making the final analysis. Mental, physical, and neurological assessments such as CAT scans, electroencephalography, and psychological tests can all be used to help determine if any other cause can be identified with the patient's symptoms. Researchers are looking for other definitive diagnostic procedures, but none has yet been discovered.

Treatment and Care

There is still no known cure for Alzheimer's disease, but proper medical care can help to minimize the effects of the disease. The victim need not be hospitalized, but must be constantly monitored by a physician. The doctor should be able to constantly measure the progression of the disease and to treat any complications that arise as a result of the problems of Alzheimer's. In addition to proper medical care and observation, some drug therapies have been effective with Alzheimer's patients. While they do not cure the disease, they can lessen the anxiety, agitation, and unpredictable behavior of the patient. A few experimental drugs that improve memory retention are also being tested. It is possible that a pill to help Alzheimer's victims retain their mental functions will be on the market at some point in the not too distant future.

The day-to-day life of the patient should also be kept as constant as possible. A regular daily routine including physical activity and social contacts will help the patient to continue functioning as normally as possible and living a normal life pattern. Proper diet and nutrition are important because many Alzheimer's victims forget how to prepare meals or even how to eat. The victim should be kept in a home-like environment as long as possible, but most patients are institutionalized as the disease progresses.

Causes of Alzheimer's Disease

Like a cure, the precise causes of Alzheimer's disease are not yet known. Many theories have identified possible factors associated with Alzheimer's disease, but none has been positively identified. One of the most likely possibilities is a change in the chemical processes of the brain. Researchers have identified a significant decrease in the activity of the cholinergic system in the brain tissues of Alzheimer's patients. Scientists are comparing Alzheimer's disease to other known syndromes in which a change in brain chemistry is implicated, such as Parkinson's disease. Unfortunately, attempts to increase the activity of the brain through chemical stimulation have not yet been successful. These chemical studies may eventually lead to a drug therapy to help Alzheimer's patients minimize the effects of the disease.

Other researchers are studying the relationship between trace metals such as aluminum and zinc and the development of the neurofibrillary tangles. Patients who have died of Alzheimer's disease have been shown to have ten to thirty times the normal concentration of aluminum in the brain. Ninety percent of the nerve cells exhibiting tangles have also been shown to contain aluminum, whereas normal nerve cells show no aluminum. While aluminum is definitely implicated in Alzheimer's disease, scientists do not know how aluminum reaches the brain or how it reacts with brain tissue. Research is currently underway to determine the normal concentrations of various trace elements in the brains of healthy individuals at all age levels so that comparisons with Alzheimer's victims may be made.

Some evidence has also been found that implies that Alzheimer's disease is hereditary. Most cases are clustered within family groups, indicating a genetic factor in the disease. One study found that relatives of Alzheimer's patients are 4.3 times as likely to contract the disease as the general population and another indicated that Alzheimer's family members are also at risk for other genetic diseases, such as Down's syndrome and leukemia. While a genetic link has been implicated, family members should be reassured that this relationship is very weak and that it does not imply that other family members will also become Alzheimer's victims.

Another possible cause of Alzheimer's disease is a slow-acting virus. Other diseases with similar symptoms, such as Creutzfeldt-Jakob disease, scrapie, and kuru, are known to be caused by transmittable viruses. Although a virus remains a possible cause of Alzheimer's, there is no evidence that Alzheimer's disease can be transmitted from one person to another. There is no danger of caretakers, health care workers, or others in contact with Alzheimer's disease patients also contracting the disease.

Psychosocial Factors of Alzheimer's Disease

One of the unfortunate tragedies of Alzheimer's disease is that it affects not only the victim, but also his/her family, friends, coworkers, and associates. Family members and other caregivers must take on the overwhelming burden of caring for the patient. This involves the constant monitoring of the patient as well as the discouragement of watching a formerly independent person lose control of his/her life. Caregivers can become extremely frustrated and depressed when the patient cannot even remember where they are or who is talking to them. Many support groups have been established for both the patients and their families. These benefit the patient by providing socialization activities and benefit the caregivers by allowing them to discuss common feelings and problems and by helping each other cope with the situation. Alzheimer's disease is also a tremendous financial burden which government programs such as medicare and medicaid do not adequately cover. Some families break under this pressure, but most find some way to persevere and care for the victims.

The Future of Alzheimer's Disease

While scientists search for the cause and a cure for Alzheimer's disease, education of the public is essential so that society will understand and assist its victims. Patients should be treated with understanding and compassion until they progress to a stage where institutionalization is necessary. We must remember that this condition is not a normal result of the aging process and that Alzheimer's disease is a terrifying illness for both its victims and their families. As more research is done on the effects and symptoms of Alzheimer's disease, both its victims and their caregivers can only hold their breath and hope for the discovery of the cause, a cure, and an effective treatment.

David A. Tyckoson
Iowa State University
October 1986

Alzheimer's Disease

1. Albert Einstein College of Medicine. Alzheimer's Disease Center. <u>Alzheimer's Disease: Questions and Answers</u>. Washington, D.C.: Government Printing Office, 1980. 12p. Superintendent of Documents Number HE20.3852:A19.
    A concise description of Alzheimer's disease, including its symptoms, diagnosis, causes, treatment, and recent research. A glossary of terms related to the disease is provided.

2. "Alzheimer's Disease: Unveiling the Mystery." <u>University of Michigan. Division of Research, Development, and Administration. The Research News</u>, v. 34, October/November 1983, pp. 12-15.
    In the many years which have passed since the German physician Alois Alzheimer identified the dementia named after him, no reliable means of conclusively diagnosing Alzheimer's disease has been developed except through autopsy. A number of University of Michigan scientists are working to devise some alternative methods of diagnosis and treatment.

3. Blass, John P. "Alzheimer's Disease." <u>DM, Disease a Month</u>, v. 31, April 1985, pp. 1-69.
    An overview of Alzheimer's disease from self-assessment questionnaires to caring for Alzheimer's victims. The widespread recognition of the importance of Alzheimer's has had some inevitable drawbacks, such as the exploitation of patients and their families and the use of Alzheimer's as an excuse for ageism.

4. Charles, Lamona, Margaret L. Truesdell, and Edna L. Wood. "Alzheimer's Disease: Pathology, Progression, and Nursing Process." <u>Journal of Gerontological Nursing</u>, v. 8, February 1982, pp. 69-73.
    The three stages and symptoms of Alzheimer's disease are detailed. Since a professional nurse is usually the primary caregiver and often the first professional person to observe changes in the patient, the nurse should be aware of current research and should keep everyone involved informed about changes in the victim.

5. Clark, Matt et al. "A Slow Death of the Mind." *Newsweek*, v. 104, December 3, 1984, pp. 56-62.
   An overview of symptoms, diagnosis, care, and research on Alzheimer's disease.

6. David, Lester and Irene David. "The Mist Lifts." *Health*, v. 17, February 1985, pp. 67-68+.
   Statistics and basic facts about the disease are presented along with some recent research results. When dealing with Alzheimer's disease, families should make sure that the attending physician is both knowledgable and attentive, that the patient follows a regular dietary routine, and that the caregivers establish a support network.

7. Duara, Ranjan and Barbara C. Black. "Report of a Statewide Conference of Scientific Investigators of Senile Dementia and Alzheimer's Disease Sponsored by the Governor of Florida." *Journal of Applied Gerontology*, v. 3, December 1984, pp. 206-213.
   The report of the first statewide conference on Alzheimer's disease from the state with the largest percentage of older adults. Among other topics discussed is the establishment of a statewide network for the exchange of information about the disease.

8. Edwards, Diane E. "A Common Medical Denominator." *Science News*, v. 129, January 25, 1986, pp. 60-62.
   Alzheimer's disease and Down's syndrome share certain neuropathological changes. This fact is helping scientists to understand both disorders and has fueled hope for new and improved treatments.

9. Emr, Marian. "Senility: The Outlook Is Bright." *World Health*, February/March 1982, pp. 13-15.
   Senility is a word that is commonly used to describe a variety of conditions. This article discusses senile dementia of the Alzheimer type (SDAT). Because of increased attention to this condition and increased funding for research, there is now more hope for its victims.

10. *Family Handbook on Alzheimer's Disease*. New York: Health Advancement Services, Inc., 1982. 24p.
    A guide for caregivers concerned with Alzheimer's disease. Topics covered include examinations to be performed before a diagnosis is accepted, the effect of the disease on the patient and the family and services available for victims.

11. Fein, Elaine. "The Fading Mind." McCall's, v. 111, August 1984, p. 47.

Alzheimer's disease steals memory and mental health. A discussion of the symptoms, types of diagnostic tests available, and programs to help both caregivers and patients.

12. Finlayson, Ann. "A Disease that Cripples the Mind." Maclean's, v. 98, June 24, 1985, pp. 48-49.

An estimated 300,000 Canadians currently suffer from Alzheimer's disease and 10,000 people died of it during the last year. The Canadian perspective on Alzheimer's is very similar to that of scientists in the United States. Researchers are frustrated with Alzheimer's research because no proven animal model exists for this disease.

13. Finn, Robert. "All About Memory." Science Digest, v. 91, November 1983, pp. 71-78.

Memory problems are a key symptom of Alzheimer's disease. Experiments to develop a drug to restore memory in Alzheimer's victims have resulted in very limited progress. Specialists caution people not to interpret every forgotten fact or incident as a symptom of Alzheimer's disease because some memory loss with age is normal.

14. Fischman, Joshua. "The Mystery of Alzheimer's." Psychology Today, v. 18, January 1984, p. 27.

An estimated 2.5 million Americans, most of them older than 65, are battling Alzheimer's disease. Scientists are struggling to learn what causes this disease and to improve techniques for diagnosis.

15. Footer, Marilyn. "Alzheimer's: Awesome Disease of the Aged." Your Life and Health, v. 98, October 1983, pp. 14-15.

Over 1.5 million Americans are suffering from Alzheimer's disease. The symptoms are becoming better defined, but diagnosis remains difficult. Causes, cures, and care are being studied, but answers are elusive.

16. Frank, Julia. *Alzheimer's Disease: The Silent Epidemics*. Minneapolis, MN: Lerner Publications, 1985. 80p. ISBN 0-8225-1578-4.

A sourcebook on Alzheimer's disease for grades five and up. Clear explanations are provided of diagnostic procedures and the effects of the disease.

17. Freedman, Gail A. "Age and Memory Loss: Myth and Reality." *Family Circle*, February 26, 1985, pp. 71-77.

Senility is widely misunderstood, particularly in its best known form, Alzheimer's disease. Scientists are now refining methods of diagnosis and treatment for senile dementia problems as well as for conditions resembling senility, such as drug intoxication and depression.

18. Goldsmith, Marsha F. "Research on Aging Burgeons As More Americans Grow Older." *JAMA: Journal of the American Medical Association*, v. 253, March 8, 1985, pp. 1369-1376+.

Life expectancy extension has included an increase in mental illness, which may mean that 45% of this country's geriatric population may develop dementia within fifty years. Since Alzheimer's disease accounts for more than one-half of all dementia cases, researchers are seeking the cause and/or cure for this disease.

19. "Growing Old." *Sciquest*, v. 53, December 1980, pp. 26-27.

Alzheimer's disease is the most common cause of intellectual impairment in persons older than sixty-five. Scientists are studying the brain, genetics, and the environment to find the causes, means of treatment, and a cure.

20. Hamilton, Harold L. "Alzheimer's Disease: The New Epidemic." <u>Nursing Homes</u>, v. 32, September/October 1983, pp. 22-26.
   A description of Alzheimer's disease, its symptoms, how a diagnosis is made, the causes and treatments, and what is being done to learn more about it. A list of definitions of terms related to Alzheimer's disease is provided.

21. Harrington-Hughes, Kathryn. "Alzheimer's Disease: As Viewed by the ACHCA." <u>Nursing Homes</u>, v. 34, January/February 1985, pp. 31-32.
   The American College of Health Care Administrators and the Alzheimer's Disease and Related Disorders Association are working together to promote awareness of and education about Alzheimer's disease. Since more than 60% of all nursing home residents are victims of Alzheimer's disease and related dementias, the ACHCA feels it is essential to educate long-term care administrators about the disease.

22. Hecht, Annabel. "Searching for Clues to Alzheimer's Disease." <u>FDA Consumer</u>, v. 19, November 1985, pp. 23-26.
   Misconceptions concerning Alzheimer's disease are still common even though it was first described nearly eighty years ago. Despite some rather predictable symptoms, Alzheimer's disease is difficult to diagnose in its early stages and a definitive diagnosis requires an autopsy. Possible causes and treatments of the disease are being studied. At this time, nothing can be done to prevent or cure Alzheimer's. Legislation has been proposed and support groups have been formed to help victims cope.

23. Heckler, Margaret M. "The Fight Against Alzheimer's Disease." <u>American Psychologist</u>, v. 40, November 1985, pp. 1240-1244.
   Some gains have been made in the United States with regard to Alzheimer's disease. Increased funding is now available for research, and support groups are becoming more readily available. There are several alternatives to institutionalization.

24. Hubbard, Linda. "The Alzheimer Puzzle: Putting the Pieces Together." **Modern Maturity**, v. 27, August/September 1984, pp. 44-47.

Only recently have public and health officials begun to recognize Alzheimer's disease as a neurological disorder distinct from the normal consequences of aging. Prominent researchers from all parts of the United States are working to uncover the cause of the disease and to develop effective diagnostic techniques and treatment methods.

25. Klumph, Leah Fackos. "Alzheimer's: Mystery Disease of the Elderly." **Editorial Research Reports**, v. 2, November 11, 1983, pp. 843-860.

Alzheimer's, a devastating and poorly understood disease, is now gaining public recognition because of its widespread occurrence among the elderly. Researchers are struggling to define the nature and extent of the disease, to find an accurate means of diagnosis, and to develop effective treatments and strategies for dealing with the problem.

26. Kvale, James N. "Alzheimer's Disease." **American Family Physician**, v. 34, July 1986, pp. 103-110.

An examination of many of the aspects of Alzheimer's disease from initial diagnosis to death, including the three stages of the disease, recommended readings, and an emphasis on concern for both the patient and the caregiver.

27. Lauter, Hans. "What Do We Know About Alzheimer's Disease Today?" **Danish Medical Bulletin**, v. 32, Supplement no. 1, February 1985, pp. 1-21.

A comprehensive review of the literature on Alzheimer's disease from epidemiology to therapy, including the importance of the psychosocial health of the caregiver.

28. Lindeman, David A. **Alzheimer's Disease Handbook**. Washington, DC: Government Printing Office, 1984. Superintendent of Documents Number HE23.3008:A19/v.1.

A comprehensive handbook on Alzheimer's disease, concentrating on the nature and scope of Alzheimer's, its psychosocial aspects, available resources and services, and family support groups.

29. Lunzer, Francesca. "Dreaded Alzheimer's." Forbes, v. 134, December 3, 1984, pp. 230-234.
   A clear, concise presentation of the facts and figures related to Alzheimer's disease. A safe, effective drug to enhance cognition would have an immediate $350 million market among Alzheimer's patients alone.

30. Martinson, Ida M. "Tell Me, Just What Am I To Do?" Journal of Gerontological Nursing, v. 10, December 1984, p. 5.
   The plight of Alzheimer's disease victims and their caregivers is examined and proposals are made through which health care professionals can help.

31. Mayeux, Richard and Wilma G. Rosen. The Dementias. New York: Raven Press, 1983. 271p. ISBN 0-87055-414-X. (Advances in Neurology, v. 38.)
   A collection of research papers on the major advances in the biological, psychological, and social aspects of dementia, including the differentiation between depression and dementia.

32. McGowan, Alan. "Alzheimer's Disease." Environment, v. 24, December 1982, p. ii.
   More funding is needed not only to find a cure for Alzheimer's disease, but also as a long term health care investment.

33. Mercer, Marilyn. "How to Tell the Difference Between Senility and Alzheimer's." Good Housekeeping, v. 200, June 1985, pp. 20+.
   Severe senile dementia affects nearly five percent of all persons over sixty-five, but only half of these have the form known as Alzheimer's disease. Strokes, Huntington's disease, and Parkinson's disease can cause other forms of senile dementia. Treatable conditions with Alzheimer-like symptoms include overmedication, malnutrition, depression, and alcoholism.

34. "The Mystery of Alzheimer's Disease." U.S. News and World Report, v. 95, Novermber 21, 1983, p. 27.
   President Reagan has proclaimed November 1983 to be National Alzheimer's Disease Month. Many articles have been written similar to this one to educate the public about the disease and its symptoms, causes, and treatments.

35. Powell, Lenore S. "Alzheimer's Disease: A Practical, Psychological Approach." *Women and Health*, v. 10, Summer/Fall 1985, pp. 53-62.

Alzheimer's disease is defined as a crippling, organic brain disorder involving loss of recent memory, unpredictable behavioral changes, and both intellectual and personality deterioration. Some helpful suggestions are provided for both the victim and the caregiver.

36. Richards, Larry D. et al. "Alzheimer's Disease: Current Congressional Response." *American Psychologist*, v. 40, November 1985, pp. 1256-1261.

An overview of the legislation which has been proposed or passed by Congress concerning Alzheimer's disease. Some of the areas covered involve research funding, assistance to patients and their families, education, and long-term care.

37. Rovner, Julie. "Alzheimer's Disease: A Puzzle Unsolved." *Congressional Quarterly Weekly Reports*, v. 44, May 31, 1986, p. 1231.

Alzheimer's victims make up one-half of the 1.2 million nursing home patients in the United States and $40 billion is spent annually on medical and related care for these victims. The federal government is beginning to focus more of its attention on this disease.

38. Sargent, Marilyn. "Alzheimer's Family Conference Held." *Adamha News*, v. 11, June 1985, pp. 1+.

The May 2, 1985 conference for families of Alzheimer's victims permitted family members to hear from and respond to the leading experts on Alzheimer's disease, to review the current situation, and to emphasize what needs to be done.

39. Sargent, Marilyn. "Questions and Answers on Alzheimer's Disease." *Adamha News*, v. 10, May 1984, pp. A5-A6.

A list of questions and answers about Alzheimer's disease, including how the brain changes, how the disease is diagnosed, and some of the drugs used for treatment.

40. "Seven Part-Time Sex Goddesses Make Like Rita Hayworth to Raise Funds for Alzheimer's Research." People, v. 24, July 29, 1985, p. 48.

April Howard, an admirer of Rita Hayworth, the actress who has Alzheimer's disease, founded the International Rita Hayworth Fan Club. Members of this club raise money for the national Alzheimer's association by dressing and singing as Rita Hayworth.

41. Shodell, Michael. "The Clouded Mind." Science 84, v. 5, October 1984, pp. 68-72.

Alzheimer's disease has become one of the most feared and devastating possibilities for the aged. It afflicts roughly five percent of the population over sixty-five, and it has no known cause, prevention, or cure. Seeking its causes and cures presents a dramatic challenge for medical researchers.

42. "Solving Mysteries of Dementia." USA Today, v. 111, February 1983, p. 11.

Since symptoms of Alzheimer's disease vary greatly among individuals, it is a difficult disease to diagnose. Although there is as yet no cure, the condition can be treated and the management of the disease is likely to improve in the future.

43. Steel, Knight and Patricia P. Barry. "Geriatrics." JAMA: Journal of the American Medical Association, v. 254, October 25, 1985, pp. 2286-2287.

With an increasingly aging population and the necessity to pay special attention to their illnesses (such as Alzheimer's), the importance of geriatric medicine is gaining more recognition. Its role is expanding into the middle years to address early control of risk factors for diseases that appear in later years.

44. Thomas, Lewis. "On the Problems of Dementia." Discover, v. 2, August 1981, pp. 34-35.

Large private foundations in the health care field should fund the needed research on dementia because they are the only hope for getting the research performed on a scale appropriate to the problem.

45. Tolliver, Lennie-Marie. "Commissioner's Corner." Aging, no. 347, 1984, p. ii.

The U.S. Commissioner on Aging presents an overview of Alzheimer's disease in her last column before her resignation.

46. Toseland, Ronald W. et al. "Alzheimer's Disease and Related Disorders: Assessment and Intervention." <u>Health and Social Work</u>, v. 9, Summer 1984, pp. 212-226.

   An overview of organic brain syndromes, effective assessment techiques, and successful methods of intervention. The benefits of early intervention by social workers is also discussed.

47. Trafford, Abigail and Joseph Carey. "Behind Spreading Fear of Two Modern Plagues." <u>U.S. News and World Report</u>, v. 99, August 12, 1985, pp. 46-47.

   Alzheimer's and AIDS are becoming the modern day equivalents of plagues of the past such as cholera or Black Death. Both are baffling to medical science and are almost always fatal. So far, Alzheimer's disease is receiving less attention in the form of research funds and appears to be an even tougher disease to deal with than AIDS.

48. U.S. Congress. House of Representatives. Select Committee on Aging. <u>Senility: The Last Sterotype</u>. Washington, DC: Government Printing Office, 1983. 94p. Superintendent of Documents Number Y4.Ag4/2:Se5/5.

   This congressional hearing was held to debunk the idea that senility is a natural consequence of aging. However, the elderly who do suffer from an irreversible dementia such as Alzheimer's disease must be helped. The difficulty in diagnosing Alzheimer's and the needs for biomedical and behavioral research are emphasized.

49. U.S. Congress. House of Representatives. Select Committee on Aging. Subcommittee on Health and Long-Term Care. <u>Alzheimer's Disease: An Information Paper</u>. Washington, DC: Government Printing Office, 1984. 61p. Superintendent of Documents Number Y4.Ag4/2:Al9/2.

   A hearing on the nature of Alzheimer's disease, its progression, diagnosis, possible causes, treatments, and financial impacts. A guide for caregivers is included.

50. U.S. Department of Health and Human Services. Task Force on Alzheimer's Disease. <u>Alzheimer's Disease: Report of the Secretary's Task Force on Alzheimer's Disease</u>. Washington, DC: Government Printing Office, 1984. 107p. Superintendent of Documents Number HE20.8102:A19/2.

    In 1983, Secretary of Health and Human Services Margaret Heckler established a departmental task force on Alzheimer's disease. The report of that study addresses nine main areas relevant to Alzheimer's and presents recommendations from leading authorities on the disease.

51. U.S. National Institute of Mental Health. Center for Studies of the Mental Health of the Aging. <u>Fact Sheet: Senile Dementia (Alzheimer's Disease)</u>. Rockville, MD: Department of Health, Education, and Welfare, Public Health Service, Alcohol, Drug Abuse, and Mental Health Administration, 1980. 4p. (DHEW Publication no. (ADM)80-929)

    Senile dementia is not a natural part of aging. This document describes Alzheimer's disease and other disorders that may be confused with it. Three federal institutes have collaborated in developing new programs for Alzheimer's victims.

52. Wallis, Claudia et al. "Slow, Steady and Heartbreaking: Alzheimer's Disease Is a Devastating Illness of Advancing Age." <u>Time</u>, v. 122, July 11, 1983, pp. 56-57.

    Although Alzheimer's disease was first identified in 1906 by the German physician Alois Alzheimer, little has been accomplished since that time to facilitate either diagnosis or treatment. While physicians can now prolong the lives of Alzheimer's victims, little has been done to improve the quality of their lives. Considerable current emphasis is directed toward improving the quality of life for both the patients and their families.

53. Wertheimer, Jean and Maurice, Marois. <u>Senile Dementia: Outlook for the Future</u>. New York: Alan R. Liss, Inc., 1984. 532p. ISBN 0-845-12305-X. (Modern Aging Research v. 5)

    Since senile dementia is a worldwide problem, it must receive worldwide attention. This volume, based on an international conference, covers all aspects of senile dementia including its socio-political connotations.

Symptoms and Causes of Alzheimer's Disease

54. "Educated Guess." <u>SciQuest</u>, v. 54, April 1981, p. 25.

It is hypothesized that a zinc deficiency may be the cause of senile dementia in patients genetically at risk for Alzheimer's disease. The administration of additional zinc could prevent or delay the onset of dementia.

55. French, L. Ronald. "A Case-Control Study of Dementia of the Alzheimer Type." <u>American Journal of Epidemiology</u>, v. 121, March 1985, pp. 414-421.

Although the exact cause of Alzheimer's disease is unknown, three possibilities involve viral, genetic, and immunologic factors. In a study of 78 Alzheimer's victims, no evidence was found to support any of these theories. A possible link between head injury and Alzheimer's was seen.

56. Grady, Denise. "Clues from Genetics and the Chemistry of the Brain May Help Solve Alzheimer's Deadly Mystery." <u>People</u>, v. 23, May 20, 1985, p. 134.

Genetic links to Alzheimer's disease include the fact that all individuals with Down's syndrome develop Alzheimer's and about one-half of all Alzheimer's cases cluster in families. A method of applying genetic engineering techniques to the analysis of the brains of Alzheimer's victims should enable scientists to locate the defective gene and discover what causes the disease.

57. Gray, Anne. "Old Before Their Time." <u>Nursing Mirror</u>, v. 154, January 13, 1982, pp. 30-32.

If there are genetic factors in Alzheimer's disease, it should be possible to screen family members for potential victims. Until then, patients with irreversible brain damage should not be placed in psychiatric hospitals, but in a hospice type setting.

58. Jenike, Michael A. "Monoamine Oxidase Inhibitors As Treatment for Depressed Patients with Primary Degenerative Dementia (Alzheimer's Disease)." <u>American Journal of Psychiatry</u>, v. 142, June 1985, pp. 763-764.

Doctors sometimes fail to treat depression in Alzheimer's patients because they consider it inevitable or untreatable. Two cases in which monoamine oxidase inhibitors were used to relieve depression are presented.

59. Kent, Saul. "What Causes Alzheimer's?" Geriatrics, v. 38, February 1983, pp. 33-41.

Although Alzheimer's disease is the most common cause of senility, scientists have been unable to identify its exact causes. Slow-acting viruses and aluminum have been among the suspected factors. Perhaps the increased research being focused on Alzheimer's will soon yield definite causes.

60. MacDonald, Donald Ian. "Protein in Brains with Alzheimer's Disease." JAMA: Journal of the American Medical Association, v. 255, June 20, 1986, p. 3217.

The discovery of a protein in the brain of Alzheimer's disease victims which is not found in normal brain tissue may shed light on the causes of this disease.

61. Mahendra, Bala. Dementia: A Survey of the Symptoms of Dementia. Boston, MA: Kluwer Academic Press, 1984. 221p. ISBN 0-85200-963-5.

Provides a critical account of the more important aspects of dementia, including clinical features, testing, management of the patient, and the historical background of the disease.

62. Mortimer, James A. and Leonard M. Schuman. The Epidemiology of Dementia. New York, Oxford University Press, 1981. 187p. ISBN 0-19-502906-2.

Based partly on a symposium on Alzheimer's disease, this volume surveys issues in the epidemiology and etiology of dementing illnesses, including methodological problems and suggestions for future research.

63. National Institute on Aging Task Force. "Senility Reconsidered: Treatment Possibilities for Mental Impairment in the Elderly." JAMA: Journal of the American Medical Association, v. 244, July 18, 1980, pp. 259-263.

The Task Force discusses the symptoms of dementia and delirium, causes, diagnostic procedures, and treatments. Reversible and irreversible brain diseases are difficult to recognize and distinguish.

64. Nee, Linda. "Studying the Family." <u>Geriatric Nursing</u>, v. 6, May/June 1985, pp. 154-156.

A study of the relationship between family history and the incidence of Alzheimer's disease showed that 75% of the study group had experienced unusual stress in the family of origin. The roles of genetically determined stress factors and inherited genes in Alzheimer's disease are stressed.

65. "A New Clue to Alzheimer's." <u>Science 84</u>, v. 5, March 1984, p. 14.

Amyloid, a substance found in the brains of Alzheimer's victims, was thought to be a waste product. A neurologist has recently discovered that it may be a prion and thus may be the cause of the disease. An analysis of the molecule could verify this result, but may take years to conduct.

66. Nolen, William A. "The Enigma of Alzheimer's: A Devastating Brain Disease Has Doctors Baffled." <u>50 Plus</u>, v. 23, August 1983, pp. 39-41.

Describes how Alzheimer's disease affects the everyday life of an individual in the early stages of the disease. At first the symptoms may be very little different than everyday forgetfulness, but as the disease progresses there is a marked deterioration of mental capacity.

67. Reisberg, Barry. "Stages of Cognitive Decline." <u>American Journal of Nursing</u>, v. 84, February 1984, pp. 225-228.

The clinical characteristics of the seven levels of cognitive function are described. For each level of cognitive decline, the patient response, impact on the family, and suggestions for professional care are given.

68. "Research Continues on the Role of Aluminum in Alzheimer's Disease." <u>Aging</u>, no. 339, May/June 1983, p. 39.

Research is continuing on the role of aluminum in the development of Alzheimer's disease.

69. Rosenfeld, Isadore. "Never Stop Hoping: It May Not Be Alzheimer's Disease." <u>Woman's Day</u>, March 4, 1986, pp. 46+.

Although Alzheimer's disease is a terrifying irreversible illness, not all signs of dementia are due to this disease. Some may be caused by other treatable conditions.

70. Storandt, Martha. "Understanding Senile Dementia: A Challenge for the Future." International Journal of Aging and Human Development, v. 16, 1983, pp. 1-6.

A review of dementia, including characteristic structural changes in Alzheimer's and treatment issues. The hypothesis that Alzheimer's is actually accelerated aging is discussed.

71. Terry, Robert D. "Some Unanswerable Questions About the Mechanisms and Etiology of Alzheimer's Disease." Danish Medical Bulletin, v. 32, Supplement no. 1, February 1985, pp. 22-24.

Questions dealing with the mechanisms of Alzheimer's disease and the ultimate cause of the disorder are presented. No answers are given, but it is hoped that useful experimental procedures will be suggested. Only laboratory research can reduce the magnitude of this problem disorder.

72. Trubo, Richard. "The Senility Virus." Science Digest, v. 89, August 1981, pp. 124-125.

Researchers suspect that certain forms of Alzheimer's disease may be caused by a virus. Sufficient evidence suggests this possibility warrants continued study.

73. U.S. Congress. House. Select Committee on Aging. Subcommittee on Human Services. Alzheimer's Disease: Is There an Acid Rain Connection? Washington, DC: Government Printing Office, 1983. 89p. Superintendent of Documents Number Y4.Ag4/2:A19.

Many of the issues surrounding the tragedy of Alzheimer's disease are examined, including the contention that acid rain may be a contributing factor. Acid rain increases the level of aluminum in the environment and aluminum can be toxic to both plant and animal life.

74. U.S. National Institutes of Health. The Dementias: Hope Through Research. Washington, DC: Government Printing Office, 1981. 32p. Superintendent of Documents Number HE20.3502:D39.

A brochure presenting an overview of dementing disorders, including research areas and the role of caregivers.

75. "Untangling the Cause." <u>Economist</u>, v. 287, April 30, 1983, pp. 112-115.

Describes the nerve pathways in dementia. Alzheimer's disease results in large part from the death of cholinergic nerve cells in parts of the brain. Unfortunately, the administration of drugs to activate cholinergic transmission have proven disappointing for unknown reasons.

76. Wurtman, Richard. "Alzheimer's Disease." <u>Scientific American</u>, v. 252, January 1985, pp. 62-66+.

In an attempt to transform Alzheimer's disease from a disease that can only be described into one that is understood and treatable, scientists are focusing on different conceptual models. They are asuming for the purpose of investigation that Alzheimer's has its origins in genetics, protein accumulation, infection, a toxin, a neurochemical disturbance, or a vascular deficiency.

77. Wyngaarden, James B. "Risk Factors for Alzheimer's Disease." <u>JAMA: Journal of the American Medical Association</u>, v. 255, March 7, 1986, p. 1105.

In a case-control study, scientists found two factors that were significantly associated with Alzheimer's disease: history of dementia among first and second degree relatives and birth to mothers older than forty years of age. However, it is emphasized that this does not necessarily mean that dementia is genetically transmitted.

Diagnosis

78. "Alzheimer's Disease." <u>American Family Physician</u>, v. 33, March 1986, pp. 347-348.

The brains of Alzheimer's victims contain less corticotropin releasing factor (CRF) and more CRF receptors than the normal brain. This discovery may be used in the future as a means of diagnosing Alzheimer's disease.

79. Carnes, Molly. "Diagnosis and Management of Dementia in the Elderly." <u>Physical and Occupational Therapy in Geriatrics</u>, v. 3, Summer 1984, pp. 11-24.

Although dementia becomes more common with age, it is not a normal part of aging. The diagnosis and possible causes of the different types of dementias are described, particularly that associated with Alzheimer's disease.

80. Cummings, Jeffrey L. et al. "Aphasia in Dementia of the Alzheimer's Type." <u>Neurology</u>, v. 35, March 1985, pp. 394-397.

A study was conducted with thirty Alzheimer's patients who were aphasic (i.e., who had either a loss or an impairment in their ability to use words). Aphasia might be used as one of the important diagnostic criteria for Alzheimer's disease.

81. Demak, Richard. "Alzheimer's Remains a Disease Beyond Diagnosis." <u>Discover</u>, v. 6, August 1985, p. 84.

Researchers have discovered some of the things that can go wrong in the brains of Alzheimer's victims, but until the cause of the disease is known there can be no direct diagnosis or cure. Scientists are investigating hereditary factors as well as the viruses and/or prions that cause scrapie and Creutzfeldt-Jacob disease.

82. Dickstein, Emil S. "Misdiagnosis of Alzheimer's Disease." <u>Geriatrics</u>, v. 37, January 1982, pp. 155-162.

In the elderly, toxic psychoses from anticholinergic drugs can be very similar to the organic brain syndrome produced by Alzheimer's disease. This fact must be kept in mind whenever a diagnosis is made.

83. Edwards, Henry. <u>What Happened to My Mother</u>. New York: Harper and Row, 1981. 175p. ISBN 0-06011-088-0.

The case study of a woman who was misdiagnosed as having Alzheimer's disease. Many months of anguish passed for both the victim and the family until she was correctly diagnosed as suffering from a treatable depression.

84. Filinson, Rachel. "Diagnosis of Senile Dementia of the Alzheimer's Type: The State of the Art." <u>Clinical Gerontologist</u>, v. 2, Summer 1984, pp. 3-23.

Diagnostic practices used for Alzheimer's disease are not sufficiently accurate. Further attempts to identify and perfect diagnostic methods are necessary, along with the further use of postmortem autopsy to confirm the presence and severity of the disease in its victims.

85. Folstein, Marshal F. and John C. S. Breitner. "Language Disorders Predict Familial Alzheimer's Disease." <u>Johns Hopkins Journal</u>, v. 149, October 1981, pp. 145-147.

The parents and siblings of Alzheimer's patients with aphasia or agraphia have a high risk of contracting the disease. Familial Alzheimer's disease is the most frequent cause of dementia seen in clinical practice.

86. "Fingerprints a Clue to Senility." <u>Science Digest</u>, v. 91, November 1983, p. 91.

A neurologist at New York University has discovered that a certain fingerprint pattern seems to occur three times as often among Alzheimer's victims as among other patients. This finding may become useful as a confirming test for senile patients whose specific diagnosis is uncertain.

87. Friedland, Robert P. et al. "The Diagnosis of Alzheimer-Type Dementia." <u>JAMA: Journal of the American Medical Association</u>, v. 252, November 16, 1984, pp. 2750-2752.

Alzheimer's disease cannot currently be diagnosed except by exclusion. Two recent techniques used to study dementia are positron emission tomography (PET) and magnetic resonance (MR) imaging. A comparative study was done of the PET and MR methods on two Alzheimer's patients.

88. Golden, Robert R., Jeanne A. Teresi, and Barry J. Gurland. "Detection of Dementia and Depression Cases with the Comprehensive Assessment and Referral Evaluation Interview Schedule." <u>International Journal of Aging and Human Development</u>, v. 16, 1982-1983, pp. 241-254.

    The Comprehensive Assessment and Referral Evaluation technique was used to collect data from two large survey groups in order to develop two indicator scales for the general detection of dementia and the detection of dementia for individuals aged sixty-five or over who are living in the community.

89. Price, Donald L. et al. "Alzheimer's Disease." <u>Annual Review of Medicine</u>, v. 36, 1985, pp. 349-356.

    Loss of memory, language disorders, and perceptual distortions are among the usual symptoms of Alzheimer's disease. Because these symptoms also appear in other treatable conditions, a correct diagnosis is crucial.

90. Reisberg, Barry. "Alzheimer's Disease Update." <u>Psychiatric Annals</u>, v. 15, May 1985, pp. 319-322.

    A global distortion scale (GDS) is presented for age-associated cognitive decline and Alzheimer's disease. The functional assessment stages and the GDS can be used by physicians and scientists to measure the amount of impairment in Alzheimer's victims.

91. Sabin, Thomas D. et al. "Are Nursing Home Diagnoses and Treatment Adequate?" <u>JAMA: Journal of the American Medical Association</u>, v. 248, July 16, 1982, pp. 321-322.

    A study of 136 nursing home patients was conducted to evaluate the potential reversibility of their neurobiological syndromes. Further investigations are necessary and there needs to be a more effective educational campaign aimed at physicians who work with the elderly.

92. Shutterworth, E. C. "Atypical Presentations of Dementia of the Alzheimer's Type." <u>Journal of the American Geriatrics Society</u>, v. 32, July 1984, pp. 485-490.

Alzheimer's disease can only be diagnosed by exclusion or autopsy, but clinical examination schemes applied to dementia patients have resulted in wide variations in neurological findings. As atypical examples, seven patients who eventually met established criteria for dementia of the Alzheimer's type are described.

93. Whall, Ann. "Alzheimer's Disease and Depression." <u>Journal of Gerontological Nursing</u>, v. 11, March 1985, p. 33.

Since Alzheimer's disease is usually diagnosed by excluding other possibilities, depression may be overlooked as a cause of the patient's disorder. Depression has symptoms similar to Alzheimer's, but the key difference is that depression can often be treated effectively. Correct diagnosis is essential to appropriate treatment of either disorder.

Care and Treatment

94. Almind, Gert. "The General Practitioner and the Dementia Patient." Danish Medical Bulletin, v. 32, Supplement no. 1, February 1985, pp. 65-67.

The general practitioner is important because he/she sees the patients and their problems at an early stage. Objectives for the care of the elderly, including dementia patients, cover the problems of the correct diagnosis of dementia (reversible or irreversible), treatment, and supplementing the care given by family members.

95. "Alzheimer's." Emergency Medicine, v. 14, September 30, 1982, pp. 187-197.

Based on interviews with researchers, the progress that has been made in understanding Alzheimer's disease is reported. The importance of excluding other causes of dementia is stressed. If the identification is Alzheimer's, the emotional and financial burden that will be placed upon the family is discussed.

96. Arrington, Carl. "A Calamity to the Victim and Family, Alzheimer's Yields Slowly to New Facilities and Medical Science." People, v. 23, May 20, 1985, pp. 122-130.

Alzheimer's victims often have been unable to get into nursing homes or to receive proper care when in them, but the Desert Life Health Care Center near Tucson has launched a successful pioneering program of care for Alzheimer's. Begun in 1979, it is being used as a model for a group of thirteen Alzheimer's homes in the west and midwest.

97. Berger, Eugene Y. "The Institutionalization of Patients with Alzheimer's Disease." Nursing Homes, v. 34, November/December 1985, pp. 22-29.

Alzheimer's is a progressive disease, almost always requiring institutionalization of its victims in the later stages. Few families acknowledge this fact and view the inevitable as a failure when it occurs. Too little emphasis is focused on the predicament of caring for Alzheimer's patients because of the preoccupation with the illness per se.

98. Brown, Dorothy S. <u>Handle with Care: A Question of Alzheimer's</u>. Buffalo, NY: Prometheus Books, 1984. 120p. ISBN 0-87975-272-6.

The author of this book cared for her mother who had Alzheimer's for ten years. Topics covered include symptoms, home care, nursing homes, and financial and legal matters for both individuals with the disease and the families that are caring for them.

99. Buys, Donna. "Slowing Down Senility." <u>Health</u>, v. 14, January 1982, pp. 16-17.

The drug THA, which has been in existence for decades, is now being used on Alzheimer's patients. THA does not stop the progression of the disease, but enhances the function of the remaining brain cells. This improves memory until so many brain cells are lost that memory impairment again becomes a problem.

100. "California Hospital Opens Alzheimer's Assessment Center." <u>Aging</u>, v. 342, December 1983/January 1984, pp. 32-33.

The Long Beach Community Hospital has created a special outpatient facility to promote a better understanding of Alzheimer's disease and to establish a pool of resources for patients, families, and private physicians.

101. Cohen, Donna and Carl Eisdorfer. <u>The Loss of Self: A Family Resource for the Care of Alzheimer's Disease and Related Disorders</u>. New York: W. W. Norton, 1986. 381p. ISBN 0-39302-263-3.

This book, written by two doctors experienced in treating Alzheimer's disease and related disorders, is a comprehensive resource interspersed with accounts of how families have coped with the tragedy of Alzheimer's.

102. Cohen, Donna et al. "Phases of Change in the Patient with Alzheimer's Dementia: A Conceptual Dimension for Defining Health Care Management." <u>Journal of the American Geriatrics Society</u>, v. 32, January 1984, pp. 11-15.

Effective treatment of Alzheimer's patients necessitates correctly gauging the stage of their illness. Phases discussed in this paper give a basis for formulating the correct treatment and identifying the resources needed.

103. Cox, Kim G. "Milieu Therapy." <u>Geriatric Nursing</u>, v. 6, May/June 1985, pp. 152-154.

Describes how a nursing unit was designed to help a group of eight patients in the early stages of Alzheimer's disease. The patients participate for a period of four to six months and have at least one family member working with them.

104. Cutler, Neal R. and Prem K. Narang. "Drug Therapies." <u>Geriatric Nursing</u>, v. 6, May/June 1985, pp. 160-163.

Among the drug therapies which have been used to treat the symptoms of Alzheimer's victims in the four stages of the disease are antidepressants, vasodilators, anxiolytic agents, and antipsychotics. Emerging therapy is targeted at the possible causes of the disease.

105. Folkenberg, Judy. "Nicotine: As a Medicine?" <u>Adamha News</u>, v. 10, December 1984, p. 5.

Despite the bad press accorded nicotine in recent years, it may be beneficial in alleviating some of the symptoms of Alzheimer's disease. Scientists are speculating that nicotine may compensate for the impairment of acetylcholine functioning in Alzheimer's victims.

106. Goldberg, Richard T. "Alzheimer's Disease: From Benign Neglect to Community Living." <u>Rehabilitation Literature</u>, v. 46, May/June 1985, pp. 122-132.

Although no means are available to reverse or stop the damage caused by Alzheimer's disease, rehabilitation techniques can be used to enable the patient to enjoy the greatest personal freedom within the constraints of his or her functional limitations.

107. Goldsmith, Marsha F. "Steps Toward Staging, Therapy of Dementia." <u>JAMA: Journal of the American Medical Association</u>, v. 251, April 13, 1984, pp. 1812-1813+.

At a conference on senile dementia of the Alzheimer's type (SDAT), the need for accurate diagnosis, prognosis, and help for the victims and caregivers was emphasized.

108. Goodman, Gerson. "Confronting Alzheimer's at Newton-Wellesley Nursing Home." **Nursing Homes**, v. 35, March/April 1986, pp. 30-34.

The Newton-Wellesley Nursing Home in Wellesley, Massachusetts began to seek outpatients diagnosed as having Alzheimer's disease as early as 1978. The staff of this facility have become pioneers in the treatment of such persons, adapting the environment and care to take full advantage of all capabilities which the patients have retained.

109. Greene, James A. et al. "Management of Alzheimer's Disease." **Journal of the Tennessee Medical Association**, v. 78, January 1985, pp. 16-23.

A review of the management of patients with Alzheimer's disease, including tests for diagnosis, treatment of depression, the side effects of the drugs used, duties of professional caregivers, and stress avoidance. Psychiatric units should be established to deal with Alzheimer's victims.

110. Gwyther, Lisa P. and Mary Ann Matteson. "Care for the Caregiver." **Journal of Gerontological Nursing**, v. 9, February 1983, pp. 92-95+.

The early, middle, and final stages of Alzheimer's disease are discussed along with probable family reactions and some appropriate services that they can use. Nurses and social workers should be able to provide continuity or a superstructure for the caregiver throughout the illness and bereavement.

111. Haugen, Per Kristian. "Behavior of Patients with Dementia." **Danish Medical Bulletin**, v. 32, Supplement no. 1, February 1985, pp. 62-65.

Dementia patients depend on support from the environment to cope with daily activities. Effective treatment measures include methods to improve orientation ability, increase social contact, and make the environment as normal as possible. In addition to more research on Alzheimer's, better evaluation methods are needed.

112. Johnson, Jean. "Nutrition As a Factor of Mortality in Senile Dementia of the Alzheimer's Type." **Psychiatric Annals**, v. 15, May 1985, pp. 323-330.

Among the factors which complicate the care of Alzheimer's patients is the nutrition element. Their emotional state inhibits eating and decreases interest in food. Severe memory loss causes these victims to forget to eat or forget how to eat.

113. Kromm, David and Young-Hie Nahm Kromm. "A Nursing Unit Designed for Alzheimer's Disease Patients at Newton Presbyterian Manor." Nursing Homes, v. 34, May/June 1985, pp. 30-31.

A special unit for Alzheimer's patients has been designed to accomodate twenty persons in a Newton, Kansas nursing home. Features include a private dining room, an open activities and exercise room, and an indoor/outdoor loop which allows patients to wander but not get lost.

114. Mace, Nancy L. and Peter V. Rabins. The 36-Hour Day: A Family Guide to Caring for Persons with Alzheimer's Disease, Related Dementing Illnesses, and Memory Loss in Later Life. Baltimore, MD: Johns Hopkins University Press, 1981. 253p. ISBN 0-8018-2660-8.

A comprehensive, practical guide for families coping with the stress and frustration of home care for Alzheimer's disease victims in the early and middle stages of the disease. Social, medical, psychological, financial, and legal aspects are all covered.

115. Middleton, Lillian. Alzheimer's Family Support Groups: A Manual for Group Facilitators. Washington, DC: Government Printing Office, 1984. 171p. Superintendent of Documents Number HE23.3008:A19/v.3.

A practical manual written for professionals and others interested in becoming facilitators of family support groups for Alzheimer's victims. In addition to information on the disease, the role of a support group and its establishment and administration are presented.

116. Montgomery, Rhonda. Family Seminars for Caregiving: Helping Families Help. Washington, DC: U.S. Department of Health and Human Services. Administration on Aging, 1984. various pagings.

Family seminars were developed as a research and demonstration project by the Pacific Northwest Long-Term Care Center to provide information, skills, and emotional support to caregivers. This manual provides the facilitator with the necessary information to present such a seminar.

117. Ninos, Mary and Rennie Makohon. "Functional Assessment of the Patient." <u>Geriatric Nursing</u>, v. 6, May/June 1985, pp. 139-143.

Since how a patient copes in his/her environment is the basis for nursing therapy, a functional assessment of the patient's physical, psychosocial, and cognitive functioning abilities is essential. Identifying the patient's areas of control and independence is equally important for other caregivers.

118. "No Man Is an Island." <u>Nursing Times</u>, v. 77, August 19-25, 1981, pp. 1466-1468.

A staff nurse, using as an example an Alzheimer's patient and a cancer patient, advises that in order for any patient to receive total care both general and psychiatric techniques of nursing must be used.

119. Palmer, Mary Happel. "Alzheimer's Disease and Critical Care." <u>Journal of Gerontological Nursing</u>, v. 9, February 1983, pp. 86-90+.

Discusses techniques that critical care nurses can follow to ensure that the goal of returning the patients to their homes is reached with a minimal disruption of the family and deterioration in function due to hospitalization.

120. Paschke, Mary J. "Day Care Within a Community Mental Health Center." <u>Physical and Occupational Therapy in Geriatrics</u>, v. 3, Summer 1984, pp. 67-70.

A day care program run by a community mental health center for at-risk and frail elderly persons was able to offer services for Alzheimer's patients. This provides an alternative to institutionalization and helps these patients sustain the skills needed for daily independent living.

121. Peppard, Nancy R. "Alzheimer Special-Care Nursing Home Units." <u>Nursing Homes</u>, v. 34, September/October 1985, pp. 25-28.

At the present time, the nursing home industry is inadequately prepared to deal with the needs of patients suffering from Alzheimer's disease and related disorders. A special unit was developed in response to the question of how to provide proper care and management for Alzheimer's victims within a nursing home setting while also being supportive of both family and staff.

122. Powell, Lenore S. and Katie Courtice. **Alzheimer's Disease: A Guide for Families**. Reading, MA: Addison-Wesley, 1983. 294p. ISBN 0-201-06099-X.

A practical guide for families that treats the feelings of guilt, frustration, and hopelessness that caregivers often experience. It also offers advice on coping with the embarrassing physical and behavioral problems that a patient may have.

123. Rabins, Peter V. "Dementia and the Family." *Danish Medical Bulletin*, v. 32, Supplement no. 1, February 1985, pp. 81-83.

Methods of managing the problems caused by the impact of dementing illnesses on the family are discussed. Not only should research on the prevention, causes, and cures for such diseases be conducted, but we should also investigate the effects of Alzheimer's on the patient and the family.

124. Reisberg, Barry et al. "An Ordinal Functional Assessment Tool for Alzheimer's-Type Dementia." *Hospital and Community Psychiatry*, v. 36, June 1985, pp. 593-595.

A new assessment tool characterizes the aspects of Alzheimer's patients' daily functioning in terms of sixteen functional assessment stages, ranging from normal to severe dysfunction. This tool should be helpful for physicians treating Alzheimer's patients.

125. Ricci, Marilyn. "All-Out Care for an Alzheimer Patient." *Geriatric Nursing*, v. 4, November/December 1983, pp. 369-371.

A description of a program worked out for an individual Alzheimer's patient. The program was designed to maintain the victim's cognitive functioning, promote her psychological comfort, and prevent her physical decline.

126. Ringland, Elinor. **Alzheimer's Disease: From Care to Caring**. Rollingbay, WA: Healthcare Press, 1984. 98p. ISBN 0-9613775-0-X.

A manual for professional health care personnel when dealing with Alzheimer's. Guidance for interaction between the patients and their families is provided and suggestions for future improvement of nursing care are given.

127. Safford, Florence. "A Program for Families of the Mentally Impaired Elderly." Gerontologist, v. 20, December 1980, pp. 656-660.

A geriatric center in New York developed a training program for families of the mentally impaired elderly. This program benefited both the participants and the nursing home institutions.

128. Sands, Dan and Thelma Suzuki. "Adult Day Care for Alzheimer's Patients and Their Families." Gerontologist, v. 23, February 1983, pp. 21-23.

The Harbor Area Adult Care Center in California was established to provide assistance to the caregivers of Alzheimer's patients by providing day care for the patients inside the home.

129. Schafer, Susan C. "Modifying the Environment." Geriatric Nursing, v. 6, May/June 1985, pp. 157-159.

The aging research nursing service at the National Institute on Aging is responsible for the nursing care of patients with Alzheimer's disease. In this unit, the nurse adapts the physical and psychosocial surroundings to the patient rather than the reverse, which is usual hospital procedure. A number of ideas involved in modifying this hospital environment could also be used in home care.

130. Schwab, Marilyn et al. "Relieving the Anxiety and Fear in Dementia." Journal of Gerontological Nursing, v. 11, May 1985, pp. 8-15.

Describes a group program used in a nursing home for dementia patients. Four primary components were stressed: simple stretching exercises, new exercises and games, walking, and relaxation. This program increased social interaction and reduced disruptive behavior in some patients.

131. "Small, Secure, Homelike Environment Best for Alzheimer's Patients." Aging, no. 347, 1984, pp. 40-41.

A special homelike environment designed for Alzheimer's patients by the University of Michigan and the Chelsea United Methodist Nursing Home has had remarkable success.

132. Volicer, Ladislav and Lawrence R. Herz. "Pharmacologic Management of Alzheimer-Type Dementia." *American Family Physician*, v. 32, July 1985, pp. 123-128.

A discussion of the types of drugs that are used in treating the symptoms of Alzheimer's disease as well as their benefits and side-effects. However, the best approach to behavioral problems may not be pharmacologic, but identifying the source of distress and alleviating it.

133. Zachary, Ruth A. "Day Care Within an Institution." *Physical and Occupational Therapy in Geriatrics*, v. 3, Summer 1984, pp. 61-67.

Day-care for Alzheimer's patients can be effectively offered within an institution. Separating Alzheimer's patients from those with similar characteristics and communicating with the patient's family are two of the key factors.

Research on Alzheimer's Disease

134. "Alzheimer's Disease Limited to Specific Brain Lesion." Public Health Reports, v. 98, July/August 1983, p. 403.

A research team has discovered that all Alzheimer's disease patients have a specific type of brain lesion. This finding provides evidence that Alzheimer's is primarily an organic brain disease rather than a psychiatric or psychological problem.

135. Anderton, Brian. "Untangling Insoluble Filaments." Nature, v. 301, January 13, 1983, p. 109.

One of the characteristics of Alzheimer's disease is the number of neurofibrillary tangles found in the brains of victims. A description of the progress made in understanding the chemical nature of these tangles is discussed.

136. "AoA Grants Focus on Support for Families of Alzheimer's Patients." Aging, no. 352, 1986, p. 26.

In the summer of 1985, the Administration on Aging awarded grants totaling approximately $1.1 million for a dozen projects designed to help both Alzheimer's victims and their families in dealing with the overwhelming emotional and financial effects of the disease.

137. Arehart-Freichel, Joan. "Aluminum Cutback to Prevent Senility." Science News, v. 124, October 1, 1983, p. 213.

A reduction of aluminum in the diet may help to prevent senile dementia or Alzheimer's disease. Although no studies have shown that aluminum reduction can prevent senility, some scientists are trying to see if a reduction can counteract the disease in Alzheimer's patients.

138. Arehart-Freichel, Joan. "Senility: The Acetylcholine Connection." Science News, v. 120, December 12, 1981, pp. 378-379.

Alzheimer's disease patients suffer from a deficiency in acetylcholine, a chemical involved in learning and memory. Results of studies using cholinergic drugs are presented.

139. Ball, M. J. et al. "A New Definition of Alzheimer's Disease: A Hippocampal Dementia." Lancet, no. 8419, January 5, 1985, pp. 14-16.

The results of a study support the hypothesis that the decline of all higher cognitive functions in senile dementia of the Alzheimer's type is attributable to histopathological changes in the hippocampal formation. The concept that the cholinergic system always underlies the cognitive decline is questioned.

140. Besson, J. A. O. et al. "The Relationship Between Parkinson's Disease and Dementia: A Study Using Proton NMR Imaging Parameters." British Journal of Psychiatry, v. 147, October 1985, pp. 380-382.

Facts show that some victims of Parkinson's disease develop a dementia and some Alzheimer's victims develop symptoms common to Parkinson's. However, the relationship between the two diseases is unclear. This study is not conclusive, but suggests that Alzheimer's type brain changes do not necessarily occur in the dementia of Parkinson's disease.

141. Bloom, Floyd. "Brain Drugs." Science 85, v. 6, November 1985, pp. 100-101.

A review of recent brain drug discoveries which imitate the chemicals in the brain in order to try and cure diseases such as depression and Alzheimer's.

142. Butler, Robert N. "The Teaching Nursing Home." JAMA: Journal of the American Medical Association, v. 245, April 10, 1981, pp. 1435-1437.

There has been a rapid growth in the numbers of elderly in the United States, but there are a lack of professionals trained in geriatric medicine. A proposal for an academic or teaching nursing home similar to teaching hospitals is made. Since Alzheimer's patients are concentrated in nursing homes, they are virtually unrepresented in clinical research. Dementia would be one of the priorities for research in the teaching nursing home.

143. Bylinsky, Gene. "Medicine's Next Marvel: The Memory Pill." Fortune, v. 113, January 20, 1986, pp. 68-71.

Drug companies are working feverishly to develop medication which will treat memory loss. Within the next five years a pill, possibly based on an acetylcholine restorer or a nootropic, could become available for this purpose. Such a pill would not cure Alzheimer's disease, but it would alleviate one of the disabling symptoms and it could become a $1 billion per year business.

144. Check, William. "Forebrain Yields Clues to Alzheimer's Disease." JAMA: Journal of the American Medical Association, v. 249, April 15, 1983, pp. 1975-1980.

Investigators have discovered that the forebrains of Alzheimer's victims show a degeneration of the neuronal cell bodies in the nuclear basalic of Meynert.

145. Clark, Matt and Mariana Gosnell. "Alzheimer's: A New Promise." Newsweek, v. 104, October 29, 1984, p. 97.

A research team has experimented with a new and promising treatment involving four Alzheimer's patients. Using a small implantable pump, doses of the acetylcholine-enhancing drug bethanechol are administered into the patient's cerebral cortex. All but one of the patients in this study appeared to benefit from this procedure.

146. Clark, Matt and Deborah Witherspoon. "A New Clue in Alzheimer's." Newsweek, v. 102, December 19, 1984, p. 94.

The amyloid deposits in the brains of Alzheimer's victims may be prions, tiny particles of protein. Prions cause three other degenerative brain disorders: Creutzfeldt-Jakob disease, scrapie, and kuru. This discovery needs further research, but it may be a clue to the cause of Alzheimer's.

147. "Closing in for the Cure." 50 Plus, v. 24, January 1984, p. 67.

A new drug, CI-911, has been developed that seems to improve the memory of Alzheimer's patients and also improves their ability to cope with everyday tasks. Testing will be completed in 1989.

148. "Commonwealth Fund Supports Research on Alzheimer's." <u>Aging</u>, no. 335/336, January/February 1983, pp. 39-40.

The Commonwealth Fund, a private philanthropic foundation which focuses on society's long-term health care needs, awarded three five-year grants for basic research on the causes of Alzheimer's disease. In citing the reasons for these donations, many basic statistics concerning Alzheimer's are provided.

149. Corkin, Suzanne et al. <u>Alzheimer's Disease: A Report of Progress in Research</u>. New York: Raven Press, 1982. 525p. ISBN 0-89004-685-9. (Aging, v. 19)

In Alzheimer's disease, the cholinergic circuit is abnormal. If drugs are given that increase the cholinergic activity, some of the symptoms may be reversed. The diagnosis, assessment of drug treatment, and choice and dose of cholinergic agents are discussed.

150. Edwards, D. D. "On the Trail of the Alzheimer's Tragedy." <u>Science News</u>, v. 128, December 14, 1985, pp. 374-375.

Three recent discoveries in regard to Alzheimer's are reported: a marked reduction of the hormone corticotropin releasing factor (CRF) in the brains of Alzheimer's victms, a SPECT study that may lead to an earlier diagnostic tool, and a neuronal biochemistry experiment using various drugs to affect catecholamine transmission in the brain.

151. Eide, Margaret and Twyla Mueller Racz. <u>Alzheimer's Disease: Bibliography of Items Published in the 1980s</u>. Ypsilanti, MI: Eastern Michigan University Library, 1985. 75p.

A bibliogrpahy of books, general and scholarly articles, newspaper accounts, and documents relating to Alzheimer's disease.

152. Emr, Marian. "Alzheimer's Research Reveals Decreased Protein Synthesis in Diseased Brains." <u>News and Features from NIH</u>, v. 84, November 1984, p. 13.

A biochemical abnormality has been discovered that impedes production of new protein in Alzheimer brain cells. This may be one of the keys in understanding the mechanisms underlying the disease.

153. Emr, Marian. <u>Progress Report on Senile Dementia of the Alzheimer Type</u>. Washington, DC: Government Printing Office, 1981. 27p. Superintendent of Documents Number HE20.3852:Se5.

 An overview of research on Alzheimer's disease prepared for the White House Conference on Aging. The role of the National Institute on Aging in promoting research on Alzheimer's disease is included.

154. English, Dallas and Donna Cohen. "A Case-Control Study of Maternal Age in Alzheimer's Disease." <u>Journal of the American Geriatrics Society</u>, v. 33, March 1985, pp. 167-169.

 Some earlier studies suggested that a relationship exists between advanced maternal age and Alzheimer's disease. The findings of this study show no evidence to support this theory.

155. "Facets of Dementia: Research on Alzheimer's." <u>Journal of Gerontological Nursing</u>, v. 10, April 1984, pp. 38-39.

 A discussion of research needs on Alzheimer's disease as presented by six panels of leading physicians at the Research Workshop on the Diagnosis of Alzheimer's Disease.

156. Finch, Caleb E. "Alzheimer's Disease: A Biologist's Perspectives." <u>Science</u>, v. 230, December 6, 1985, p. 1109.

 How will the increased emphasis on Alzheimer's disease influence support of and opportunities for basic research? Among the possibilities is a greater availability of brain tissues from normal subjects which can be used for various types of research.

157. Fine, Alan. "Peptides and Alzheimer's Disease." <u>Nature</u>, v. 319, February 13, 1986, pp. 537-538.

 In addition to the cholinergic system, other neurotransmitters are reduced in the brains of Alzheimer's victims. The implications of this finding on the pathology of the disease are presented.

158. Fischman, Joshua. "Untangling Alzheimer's Disease." <u>Psychology Today</u>, v. 18, December 1984, p. 13.

 An important connection has been made between the location of brain damage in Alzheimer's disease and certain behavioral changes in Alzheimer's patients.

159. "Five Centers for Alzheimer's Research Established." <u>Public Health Reports</u>, v. 100, January/February 1985, p. 108.
   Five Alzheimer's disease centers have been established by the Department of Health and Human Services and are funded by grants from the National Institute on Aging. Research at the centers will be conducted according to guidelines set forth by the Alzheimer's Disease Task Force Report.

160. Folkenberg, Judy. "Preliminary Alzheimer's Findings." <u>Adamha News</u>, v. 112, March 1986, p. 7.
   Scientists at the National Institute of Mental Health have conducted research using deprenyl, an anti-depressant, to treat a group of seventeen Alzheimer's disease patients. Preliminary evidence suggests that deprenyl slightly improved mood and memory function.

161. Forsythe, Jason. "Alzheimer's and Down Syndrome: A Genetic Link?" <u>Psychology Today</u>, v. 20, March 1986, p. 9.
   Recent findings suggest a genetic link between Alzheimer's disease and Down's syndrome. However, the only proven link is that these two diseases cause strikingly similar changes in the brain.

162. Francis, Paul T. et al. "Neurochemical Studies of Early-Onset Alzheimer's Disease: Possible Influence on Treatment." <u>New England Journal of Medicine</u>, v. 313, July 4, 1985, pp. 7-11.
   The discovery of multiple neurotransmitter deficiencies in autopsy studies of Alzheimer's disease patients indicates that simple cholinergic replacement therapy may not be successful.

163. Glenner, G. G. "Alzheimer's Disease (Senile Dementia): A Research Update and Critique with Recommendations." <u>Journal of the American Geriatrics Society</u>, v. 30, January 1982, pp. 59-62.
   Reviews the research findings on Alzheimer's disease and discusses the problems involved in studying it. Some new approaches, such as enzyme and neuronal receptor studies, are recommended.

164. Goldsmith, Marsha F. "Attempts to Vanquish Alzheimer's Disease Intensify, Take New Paths." JAMA: Journal of the American Medical Association, v. 251, April 13, 1984, pp. 1805-1812.

At a conference on Alzheimer's disease, laboratory researchers described efforts to discover the cause of the disease and the need to have the brains of deceased victims for autopsy.

165. Herbert, Wray. "Senility: Sitting on a Time Bomb." Science News, v. 122, October 23, 1982, p. 270.

An analysis of family histories of Alzheimer's disease patients indicates that the disease is inheritable and that the genetic makeup for Alzheimer's is much more prevalent than previously thought. Research also shows that the most reliable indicator of familial Alzheimer's is a breakdown in linguistic ability. In an aging population, more and more dementia will be seen.

166. Hinton, David R. et al. "Optic-Nerve Degeneration in Alzheimer's Disease." New England Journal of Medicine, v. 315, August 21, 1986, pp. 485-487.

The diagnosis of Alzheimer's disease has always been one of exclusion. However, the recent discovery of the degeneration of retinal ganglion cells and of the optic nerve in patients with Alzheimer's is clearly distinguishable from the age-matched controls and could facilitate the clinical diagnosis of the disease.

167. Hutton, J. Thomas and Alexander D. Kenny. Senile Dementia of the Alzheimer Type. New York: Alan R. Liss, 1985. 404p. ISBN 0-84512-720-9.

A collection of papers based on the 1984 Norman Rockwell Conference on Alzheimer's disease which presents and consolidates recent research and treatments for Alzheimer's. Special emphasis is given to possible etiologies of Alzheimer's and to the probability that dysfunction of the blood-brain barrier may play a role.

168. Katzman, Robert. "Alzheimer's Disease." *New England Journal of Medicine*, v. 314, April 10, 1986, pp. 964-973.

A review of progress and research findings on the various aspects of Alzheimer's disease and its recognition as a major health problem.

169. Kelly, William E. *Alzheimer's Disease and Related Disorders*. Springfield, IL: Charles C. Thomas, 1984. 230p. ISBN 0-398-04895-9.

A collection of papers from a conference on Alzheimer's disease with emphasis on current research, treatment, and available programs.

170. Khachaturian, Zaven S. "Progress of Research on Alzheimer's Disease: Research Opportunities for Behavioral Scientists." *American Psychologist*, v. 40, November 1985, pp. 1251-1255.

Certain types of research in the behavioral sciences, such as longitudinal studies of Alzheimer's victims and general aged populations, might improve the diagnosis of Alzheimer's disease.

171. Kolata, Gina. "Down Syndrome-Alzheimer's Linked." *Science*, v. 230, December 6, 1985, pp. 1152-1153.

Recent studies of people with Down's syndrome and patients with Alzheimer's disease are revealing previously unexpected similarities between the two. While every Down's syndrome adult who lives beyond the age of thirty develops the brain lesions typical of Alzheimer's disease, only a few become demented. The discovery of parallels between Down's syndrome and Alzheimer's disease may open new doors in the future.

172. Levy, Raymond. "Lecithin in Alzheimer's Disease." *Lancet*, no. 8299, September 18, 1982, pp. 671-672.

The effects of lecithin on Alzheimer's dementia should not be dismissed too soon. Even a slowing down of the intellectual decline which results in a postponement of institutionalizing the patient would have significant social and financial considerations.

173. Martin, Alex et al. "On the Nature of the Verbal Memory Deficit in Alzheimer's Disease." Brain and Language, v. 25, July 1985, pp. 323-341.

The verbal memory of fourteen Alzheimer's patients was compared with eleven normal persons. Predictably, the Alzheimer patients fared worse, but the pattern of recall across conditions seemed similar. Alzheimer's memory impairment may be due mainly to an inability to encode a sufficient number of stimulus features.

174. McAuliffe, Sharon. "Genetic Time Bombs for the Elderly." Psychology Today, v. 17, May 1983, p. 21.

Research indicates that most cases of Alzheimer's disease may have genetic origins. Studying the familial form of Alzheimer's has been difficult because the dementia typically does not show up until about age eighty. With life expectancies increasing, familial Alzheimer's may become an explosive medical problem.

175. Miller, J. A. "For Want of an Inhibitor: Alzheimer's Disease." Science News, v. 126, September 1, 1984, p. 132.

Scientists have discovered that the inhibitory protein which prevents ribonuclease from destroying RNA is either absent or ineffective in Alzheimer's disease. More studies are required to determine if this is a cause or a symptom, but in any case it may lead to improvement in diagnosis and treatment.

176. Mohs, Richard C. et al. "Oral Physostigmine Treatment of Patients with Alzheimer's Disease." American Journal of Psychiatry, v. 142, January 1985, pp. 28-33.

Oral physostigmine was administered to twelve Alzheimer's patients in order to evaluate the effect of this treatment on the disease. Of the ten patients who completed the study, three showed significant improvement and four more showed marginal improvement.

177. Newell, John. "Acetylcholine, Alzheimer's, and Stomach Ulcers." New Scientist, v. 110, June 19, 1986, p. 36.

In attempting to find a compound that would make the brain of an Alzheimer's victim more sensitive to acetylcholine, approximately twenty compounds have been discovered that have the reverse effect. However, these agents could be used to quiet over responses such as too much acid produced in the stomach, leading to ulcers.

178. Pardes, Herbert. "Alzheimer's Disease: Director Reports on NIMH-Funded Research." Adamha News, v. 9, August 19, 1983, pp. 4-5.

An outline of the intensive research on Alzheimer's disease conducted and supported by the National Institute of Mental Health.

179. Reisberg, Barry. Alzheimer's Disease: The Standard Reference Book. New York: Free Press, 1983. 475p. ISBN 0-02-926230-5.

Research results emphasizing the biomedical and neuroscience aspects of Alzheimer's disease are compiled in this reference work.

180. Schneider, Edward L. and Marian Emr. "Research Highlights." Geriatric Nursing, v. 6, May/June 1985, pp. 136-138.

Research described includes work being done with neurotransmitters, protein synthesis, and slow viral diseases. Background information is provided on the aging of the American population and its relation to the growing incidence of Alzheimer's disease.

181. Scileppi, Kenneth P. et al. "Circulating Vitamins in Alzheimer's Dementia as Compared with Other Dementias." Journal of the American Geriatrics Society, v. 32, October 1984, pp. 709-711.

No significant difference was found between the vitamin blood levels of Alzheimer's victims and the control subjects. Vitamin malnutrition does not appear to contribute to the disabilities of the victims.

182. "Secretary's Alzheimer's Report." *Adamha News*, v. 10, November 1984, pp. 2-3.

A summary of the report of the Task Force on Alzheimer's Disease. Twenty-seven recommendations are made for research in seven different areas, including diagnosis, treatment, family aspects, and systems of care.

183. Shore, David et al. "Hair and Serum Copper, Zinc, Calcium, and Magnesium Concentrations in Alzheimer-Type Dementia." *Journal of the American Geriatrics Society*, v. 32, December 1984, pp. 892-895.

A report on the results of a study to detect significant differences of several minerals between Alzheimer's victims and control subjects.

184. Silberner, Joanne. "Alzheimer's Disease: Soul Searching." *Science News*, v. 128, July 13, 1985, p. 24.

Brain biopsies are only rarely done to confirm the diagnosis of Alzheimer's disease, but British researchers studied the tissue collected from seventeen patients over a five year period. They concluded that the more seriously affected the victim, the less acetylcholine was being produced.

185. "Theories and Therapies." *American Journal of Nursing*, v. 84, February 1984, pp. 223-224.

Key theories and therapies on Alzheimer's disease currently under investigation are listed with a brief description of each.

186. U.S. Congress. House. Committee on Science and Technology. Subcommittee on Investigations and Oversight. *Alzheimer's Disease*. Washington, DC: Government Printing Office, 1985. 33p. Superintendent of Documents Number Y4.Sci2:98/00.

A summary of research results on Alzheimer's disease presented to Congress. Research on health care funding and policy changes are included.

187. Wheater, R. H. "Aluminum and Alzheimer's Disease." JAMA: Journal of the American Medical Association, v. 253, April 19, 1985, p. 2288.

Although researchers have been studying the brain aluminum levels between Alzheimer's patients and control groups, results have been contradictory. It appears that although aluminum is not the sole cause, it may mark the degeneration of the neurons or Alzheimer's patients may simply be more vulnerable to the neurotoxic effects of the metal.

188. White, June A., Matthew McGue, and Leonard L. Heston. "Fertility and Parental Age in Alzheimer Disease." Journal of Gerontology, v. 41, January 1986, pp. 40-43.

A study to investigate the association between Alzheimer's disease and parental age and reduced fertility concluded that neither factor had an effect for Alzheimer's disease.

Case Studies, Clinical Reports, and Statistics

189. "Alzheimer's Disease: Thief of the Mind." *Current Health 2*, v. 2, May 1984, pp. 20-21.

Dramatic differences were seen between the brains of patients who died of Alzheimer's disease and the brains of those without the disease. Alzheimer's victims had only five percent of the normal number of nerve cells in the basal forebrain. Researchers have not yet been able to identify the causes of the disease or to develop an effective means of diagnosis.

190. Brody, Elaine M. et al. "Predictors of Falls Among Institutionalized Women with Alzheimer's Disease." *Journal of the American Geriatrics Society*, v. 32, December 1984, pp. 877-882.

Falls of the elderly can be extremely serious. The results of a study of falls among a group of patients with Alzheimer's disease are reported.

191. Crook, Thomas H. and Nancy E. Miller. "The Challenge of Alzheimer's Disease." *American Psychologist*, v. 40, November 1985, pp. 1245-1250.

A case report of a 73-year-old female Alzheimer's patient illustrates the multiple problems involved in the diagnosis and treatment of this disease.

192. Cummings, Jeffrey L. and D. Frank Benson. *Dementia: A Clinical Approach*. Boston, MA: Butterworth, 1983. 416p. ISBN 0-409-95044-0.

This reference guide takes recent research results on dementia and applies them to the clinical identification and differential diagnosis of demented patients.

193. Dalessio, Donald J. "Maurice Ravel and Alzheimer's Disease." *JAMA: Journal of the American Medical Association*, v. 252, December 28, 1984, pp. 3412-3413.

Maurice Ravel, the famous twentieth century composer, began exhibiting the symptoms of Alzheimer's disease at the age of 56. Eventually he declined into amusia, the inability to produce or comprehend musical sounds. Ravel's loss of creativity is described as one of the artistic tragedies of our times.

194. Feil, Naomi. "Communicating with the Confused Elderly Patient." Geriatrics, v. 39, March 1984, pp. 131-132.

Among the effective measures to use when communicating with a confused elderly patient are the following: establish eye contact, listen attentively, use touch, gently lead conversation from fantasy to reality, and affirm the validity of the patient's emotions.

195. Greene, James A., Jan Arp, and Nancy Crane. "Specialized Management of the Alzheimer's Disease Patient: Does It Make A Difference? A Preliminary Research Report." Journal of the Tennessee Medical Association, v. 78, September 1985, pp. 559-563.

Special management techniques for handling Alzheimer's patients have been established at the Knoxville Health Care Center. Pre- and post-evaluation of the patients show a quality of life improvement. Future plans call for comprehensive testing to ensure greater diagnostic accuracy of Alzheimer's disease.

196. Herbert, Wray. "Memory in the Rough." Psychology Today, v. 17, September 1983, p. 18.

Selected memory loss in an Alzheimer's patient was studied by playing golf with the victim. This case study and laboratory research both indicate that there may be different physiological mechanisms responsible for the different kinds of memory traces.

197. Mace, Nancy L. "Facets of Dementia: Is Alzheimer's Disease Transmissable?" Journal of Gerontological Nursing, v. 10, June 1984, p. 42.

Although Creutzfeldt-Jacob disease, a dementing illness, can be transmitted from person to person, there is no evidence that the same is true for Alzheimer's disease. A genetic risk for Alzheimer's does exist, but families should be reassured that this risk is very low.

198. Miller, Nancy E. and Gene D. Cohen. Clinical Aspects of Alzheimer's Disease and Senile Dementia. New York: Raven Press, 1981. 357p. ISBN 0-89004-326-4. (Aging, v. 15)

A collection of papers presented at the second joint conference of the National Institutes of Health and ADAMHA. All of the problems of dementia are covered, with emphasis placed on the clinical aspects of the disease, patient care, and services.

199. Miot, C. "Alzheimer's Report: Mapping Cell Damage." Science News, v. 126, September 15, 1984, p. 167.

A new staining technique has been developed that specifically dyes a substance in the nerve tangles of Alzheimer's victims. This allows the mapping of the exact sites of brain damage from Alzheimer's disease.

200. "New Hope for Alzheimer's." McCall's, v. 112, January 1985, pp. 37-38.

Alzheimer's patients suffer from a shortage of acetylcholine, which carries messages through the brain. Recent experiments with bethanechol chloride indicate that this substance may mimic the action of acetylcholine when injected into the brains of Alzheimer's patients. This is the first step toward understanding and controlling the disease.

201. Parker, Joseph C. "Alzheimer's Disease: A Major Health Problem." Journal of the Tennessee Medical Association, v. 78, January 1985, pp. 9-12.

A description of the clinical and autopsy procedures used on Alzheimer's patients. The probable causes of this disease, which is the most common neurodegenerative disorder in man, are discussed.

202. Powers, Laura B. and John H. Dougherty, Jr. "Dementia of the Alzheimer's Type: Clinical Overview." Journal of the Tennessee Medical Association, v. 78, January 1985, pp. 13-15.

A review of the definition, pathology, biochemistry, etiology, clinical presentation, and diagnosis of Alzheimer's disease. When assessing the patient, it is important to rule out the possibility of depression or pseudodementia, both of which are treatable.

203. Stern, Matthew B. et al. "Dementia of Parkinson's Disease and Alzheimer's Disease: Is There a Difference?" Journal of the American Geriatrics Society, v. 34, June 1986, pp. 475-478.

Scientific studies are not clear on the differences between dementia caused by Alzheimer's or Parkinson's disease. It appears that although Alzheimer's may coexist in some victims of Parkinson's disease, evidence points to a unique chemical disequilibrium in Parkinson's patients.

204. "Sugar Ray Robinson in Biggest Battle of Life As Holiday Season Approaches." *Jet*, v. 69, December 30, 1985, p. 50.

Sugar Ray Robinson, a boxer for over twenty-five years, is now a victim of Alzheimer's disease. He continues to serve as the director of a sports foundation bearing his name, but friends report that his attention span is minimal and that he often forgets even simple details. It is unkown if his current problems are related to his many years in the ring.

205. Tisdale. Sally. "Life As a Stream of Consciousness: Alzheimer's Disease." *CoEvolution Quarterly*, v. 43, Fall 1984, pp. 22-33.

Case studies of different Alzheimer's victims are interspersed with factual information about the causes, diagnosis, treatment, and current research on Alzheimer's disease.

206. Wisniewski, K. E. et al. "Occurrence of Neuropathological Changes and Dementia of Alzheimer's Disease in Down's Syndrome." *Annals of Neurology*, v. 17, March 17, 1985, pp. 278-282.

Victims of Down's syndrome seem to be vulnerable to early development of Alzheimer's disease. The reason for this is unknown, but many possibilities are discussed, including an immunological defect.

207. Zarit, Steven H., Judy M. Zarit, and Karen E. Reever. "Memory Training for Severe Memory Loss: Effects on Senile Dementia Patients and Their Families." *Gerontologist*, v. 22, August 1982, pp. 373-377.

The effects of memory training exercises on non-institutionalized senile dementia patients and their caregivers was studied. Although the results indicated that the clinical application of memory training appears limited, some elements of the program were of value to the caregivers, including both counseling and support groups.

Personal Narratives

208. Adamo, Jane. "What's Happened to Mother?" Good Housekeeping, v. 197, August 1983, pp. 90+.

When the author's mother began to show signs of senility at age 52, the family was baffled. When doctors made the diagnosis of Alzheimer's disease, the family made the difficult decisions necessary to cope with the situation.

209. Atkins, Marguerite Henry. Also My Journey: A Personal Story of Alzheimer's. Wilton, CT: Morehouse Barlow Co., 1985. 160p. ISBN 0-8192-1362-4.

After seven years of marriage, Dick Atkins was stricken with Alzheimer's disease and eventually was hospitalized for nine years. There were few support groups in existence at that time, but his wife was able to cope because of her love for her husband and her faith in God.

210. Barlow, A. Ralph. "Senile Dementia: Metaphor for Our Time." Christian Century, v. 100, February 16, 1983, pp. 151-153.

A description of how the author's father suffered from Alzheimer's for six years. The disease hampered the possibility that they could rediscover their affinity in the later years of their relationship.

211. Brandt, Anthony. "A Woman of Character." Esquire, v. 102, August 1984, pp. 17-18.

At age eighty, the author's mother has been a victim of Alzheimer's disease for nearly a decade. She no longer speaks intelligibly and responds to the presence of others in an unpredictable manner, yet she handles her own situation with remarkable equanimity. Her inner strength endures and she continues to teach others how to understand her misfortune.

212. Doubleday, Opal A. Whilst Thy Tower Crumbles. New York: Vantage Press, 1984. 141p. ISBN 5-3305-965-8.

The story of a man who began to show confusion and anxiety in 1966, but who was not diagnosed as a victim of Alzheimer's disease until 1975. The struggle with his disease is recounted from its beginnings until his death in 1981.

213. Ghazarbekian, Bonnie. "Mother and the Nursing Home." Reader's Digest, v. 122, June 1983, pp. 133-136.
   The story of a woman who moved her mother, who was suffering from Alzheimer's disease, from her home environment to a nursing home. The problems of caring for the elderly seem to center on three questions: What will make the aged person happiest?, What is best for the patient?, and What is best for the family?

214. Glaze, Bobbie. "One Woman's Story." Journal of Gerontological Nursing, v. 8, February 1982, pp. 67-68.
   A description of how one family coped with a man who suffered from Alzheimer's disease for twelve years. His spouse has become involved in family support groups in order to help others avoid some of the same problems.

215. Hemshorn, Agnes. "They Call It Alzheimer's Disease." Journal of Gerontological Nursing, v. 11, January 1985, pp. 36-38.
   The story of how a family coped with a man who suffered from Alzheimer's during the early stages of the disease.

216. Holland, Gail Bernice. For Sasha, With Love: An Alzheimer's Crusade. New York: Dembner Books, 1985. 192p. ISBN 0-934878-54-4.
   Two Russian emigres found the American dream in southern California until the husband was stricken with Alzheimer's disease. The bitterness and suffering they endured due to the lack of a national long-term health care plan led to the political activism of the wife and the passage of the first state-wide law in the nation to help brain-damaged adults and their families.

217. Hollister, Anne et al. "The Fading Mind: Alzheimer's Takes a Terrible Toll on the Family." Life, v. 9, February 1986, pp. 30-36+.
   Three families struggling to care for relatives afflicted with Alzheimer's disease illustrate the frustrations and heartaches involved. A day care center is highlighted. Similar programs may provide some relief and support for both the victims and their families.

218. Jarvis, J. "Now Rita Sits in Silence." People, v. 20, November 7, 1983, pp. 112-113.

Rita Hayworth, the glamorous movie star of the 1940s, is a victim of Alzheimer's disease. She can no longer speak and requires a nurse on a full time basis. Her daughter is now a national spokesperson on behalf of Alzheimer's disease.

219. Lerner, Marguerite R. "I've Lost a Kingdom: A Victim's Remarks on Alzheimer's Disease." Journal of the American Geriatrics Society, v. 32, December 1984, p. 935.

A collection of quotations from Marguerite Lerner, a former physician and children's book author who became ill with Alzheimer's disease in her mid-fifties. Her husband recorded her remarks about the disease early each morning when her thoughts were the most clear.

220. Pressler, Larry. "A Father's Senility Becomes a Losing Battle for a U.S. Senator and His Family." People, v. 18, July 12, 1982, pp. 40-43.

Senator Pressler's father, a farmer, began to show signs of forgetfullness at age 59. The family did not realize the seriousness of the disease until they learned that the father could not take care of his feeder calves. The family gradually came to grips with Alzheimer's disease and feels that it is unfair to see their father in this condition of dependency because he never wanted to be dependent on anyone.

221. Roach, Marian. Another Name for Madness. Boston, MA: Houghton Mifflin Co., 1985. 241p. ISBN 0-395-35373-4.

A biography of the author's mother, who became ill with Alzheimer's disease at the age of 51. The family had a feeling of helplessness and anguish when providing care and watching a vibrant mother descend into the senility of this devastating disease.

222. Roach, Marian. "Another Name for Madness: A Family's Losing Battle with Alzheimer's Disease." New York Times Magazine, January 16, 1983, pp. 22-23+.

The story of the author's mother, a 54 year old Alzheimer's victim. The family learned from firsthand experience the problems involved in diagnosing and coping with the early stages of the disease. This is a vivid portrayal of the nightmarish quality that life takes for both Alzheimer's victims and their families.

223. Roach, Marian. "Reflection in a Fatal Mirror." Discover, v. 6, August 1985, pp. 76-82+.

The author's mother is a 56 year old Alzheimer's victim who has had the disease for seven years. Historical and medical facts are interspersed with poignant personal experiences. The reverse devlopment theory is emphasized, which states that Alzheimer's victims become progressively more childlike as time goes by.

224. Santini, Rosemary and Katherine Barrett. "The Tragedy of Rita Hayworth." Ladies Home Journal, v. 100, January 1983, pp. 84-85+.

An interview with the daughter of Rita Hayworth about the effects of Alzheimer's disease on her mother. She has asked President Reagan for his support in fighting Alzheimer's and also highlights recent research findings about the disease.

225. Seymour, Claire. Precipice: Learning to Live with Alzheimer's Disease. New York: Vantage Press, 1983. 182p. ISBN 0-533-05619-5.

An intensely discerning and compassionate account of one woman's life with a husband who had Alzheimer's. Her faith allowed her to keep hope when dealing with a seemingly impossible situation.

226. Woodward, Joanne. "When I Go to See My Mother Now I Weep." TV Guide, May 18, 1985, pp. 17-19.

The actress Joanne Woodward writes about her mother, who apparently has contracted Alzheimer's disease. The mother is no longer able to speak or recognize her daughter.

227. Wooll, Alfred C. <u>In Sickness And In Health: A Description of One Family's Struggle with Alzheimer's Disease</u>. Ann Arbor, MI: Ann Arbor Chapter. Alzheimer's Disease and Related Disorders Association, 1985. 80p.

    An account in diary form of how one man's wife fell ill with Alzheimer's disease. The deterioration of her abilities and the care by the family is highlighted.

Psychological and Social Aspects of Alzheimer's Disease

228. "Alzheimer's Disease: Understanding Is the Only Medicine." <u>University of Michigan. Division of Research Development and Administration. Research News</u>, v. 34, October/November 1983, pp. 7-11.
   Presents the results of a study of the effects of Alzheimer's disease on the families of the victims. A number of questions are raised. Alzheimer's disease is now the fourth leading cause of death.

229. Aronson, Miriam and Elaine S. Yatzkan. "Coping with Alzheimer's Disease Through Support Groups." <u>Aging</u>, no. 347, 1984, pp. 3-9.
   The need for support groups for families of Alzheimer's disease victims is clear. A number of different types of groups are springing up in response to otherwise unfilled needs. The self-help movement is having an impact on the formal service network.

230. Aronson, Miriam et al. "A Community Based Family/Patient Group Program for Alzheimer's Disease." <u>Gerontologist</u>, v. 24, August 1984, pp. 339-342.
   Describes a program in which patients and their families meet simultaneously at a gerontology center each week. The family group helps members cope with their problems as caregivers and the patient group provides socialization activities for the victims.

231. Barnes, Robert F. et al. "Problems of Families Caring for Alzheimer's Patients: Use of a Support Group." <u>Journal of the American Geriatrics Society</u>, v. 29, February 1981, pp. 80-85.
   An eight-week support group program served as the prototype for additional programs to help families cope with home care of Alzheimer's patients. Common problems for such families include the lack of support and information from physicians, poor understanding of the disease, a trapped feeling, anger, fear, isolation, and the caretaker's loss of self-identity.

232. Berman, Stephen and Meryl B. Rappaport. "Social Work and Alzheimer's Disease: Psychosocial Management in the Absence of Medical Cure." <u>Social Work in Health Care</u>, v. 10, Winter 1984, pp. 53-70.

Because of the devastating effect that Alzheimer's disease has on the personality of its victims, both the patients and their families have a critical need for psychosocial assistance. Specific types of intervention help patients and caregivers to adapt during the usually long course of this disease.

233. "Coping with the Incurable." <u>USA Today</u>, v. 113, October 1984, pp. 7-8.

Alzheimer's disease has no known cause or cure. Some ideas for stress reduction and behavioral intervention are given to help families cope with Alzheimer's disease.

234. Crossman, Linda et al. "Older Women Caring for Disabled Spouses: A Model for Supportive Services." <u>Gerontologist</u>, v. 21, October 1981, pp. 464-470.

Among the elderly, women are the primary caregivers, often at the risk of their own health. A multi-service program was established in California to help such women. The future implications of this program are explored, especially in view of the changing roles of women in society.

235. Cybyk, M. E. "Alzheimer's Disease." <u>Nursing Times</u>, v. 76, February 14, 1980, pp. 280-282.

The three stages of Alzheimer's disease are described, along with the testing of a female patient diagnosed as having the disease. The denial reaction of her husband is examined.

236. Dilka, Carol. "Alzheimer's and Your Employees." <u>Nation's Business</u>, v. 73, April 1985, p. 68.

Some suggestions are given for businesses in helping caregiver employees cope with Alzheimer's disease in their families. These include stipends to cover medical or dependent care expenses, posting information about support groups, access to the company's legal department, and work schedule flexibility.

237. Glosser, Guila and Debra Wexler. "Participants' Evaluation of Educational/Support Groups for Families of Patients with Alzheimer's Disease and Other Dementias." Gerontologist, v. 25, June 1985, pp. 232-236.

Fifty-four participants in a seven week educational and support group evaluated the helpfulness of the different aspects of their group experience. Overall, the evaluations were positive, but the ultimate success of such programs depends on their inclusion within a much broader service network.

238. Hayter, Jean. "Helping Families of Patients with Alzheimer's Disease." Journal of Gerontological Nursing, v. 8, February 1982, pp. 81-86.

Nearly one hundred relatives of patients with Alzheimer's disease have expressed their problems and frustrations in dealing with the disease. Almost all of the families needed more help than they were getting in coping with their caretaker responsibilities. Suggestions are made for ways in which nurses can help families deal with Alzheimer's disease.

239. Hirschfeld, Miriam. "Homecare Versus Institutionalization: Family Caregiving and Senile Brain Disease." International Journal of Nursing Studies, v. 20, 1983, pp. 23-32.

In order for families to continue home care for patients with irreversible senile dementia, it is necessary for them to find gratification in their relationships with the patient.

240. Kahan, Jason et al. "Decreasing the Burden in Families Caring for a Relative with a Dementing Illness: A Controlled Study." Journal of the American Geriatrics Society, v. 33, September 1985, pp. 664-670.

Caring for an Alzheimer's patient is very stressful, both mentally and physically. In recognition of this fact, many programs are being developed to support caregivers. An eight-week support group program was examined and the effect of the program was positive, especially the educational component.

241. LaBarge, Emily. "Counseling Patients with Senile Dementia of the Alzheimer Type and Their Families." Personnel and Guidance Journal, v. 60, November 1981, pp. 139-143.

Although the emotional burden is heavy on family members of Alzheimer's victims, they do not receive enough support from the gerontology field. Some counseling techniques for family members of Alzheimer's victims are presented.

242. Lazarus, Lawrence W. et al. "A Pilot Study of an Alzheimer Patient's Relatives Discussion Group." Gerontologist, v. 21, August 1981, pp. 353-358.

During a testing program using cholinergic drugs on elderly Alzheimer patients, a study was conducted on the coping mechanisms of the relatives and the effect of a relatives discussion group. Alzheimer's patients need to be considered as members of a family network and not as a separate entity.

243. Mobily, Kenneth E. and Thea M. Hoeft. "The Family Dilemma: Alzheimer's Disease." Activities, Adaptation, and Aging, v. 6, Summer 1985, pp. 63-71.

Leisure activities can enhance the quality of life for both Alzheimer's victims and those who care for them. Recreation can be used as a medium for positive experiences, communication, and continued use of remaining abilities.

244. Oliver, Rose and Frances A. Bock. "Alleviating the Distress of Caregivers of Alzheimer's Disease Patients: A Rational-Emotive Therapy Model." Clinical Gerontologist, v. 3, Summer 1985, pp. 17-34.

Caring for Alzheimer's victims places a sizable emotional burden on the caregiver, who often responds with symptoms such as anger, denial, depression, guilt, and self-pity. Rational-emotive therapy may help these persons.

245. Pagel, Mark D., Joseph Becker, and David B. Coppel. "Loss of Control, Self-Blame, and Depression: An Investigation of Spouse Caregivers of Alzheimer's Disease Patients." Journal of Abnormal Psychology, v. 94, May 1985, pp. 169-182.

A longitudinal study was conducted of caregivers of spouses with Alzheimer's disease using the reformulated learned helplessness (RLH) depression model. Caregiver depression levels were predicted at current and ten-month followup periods.

246. Panella, John J. et al. "Day Care for Dementia Patients: An Analysis of a Four-Year Program." *Journal of the American Geriatrics Society*, v. 32, December 1984, pp. 883-886.

Although day care programs can not halt or change the intellectual decline of dementia patients, it does provide respite time for the caregivers. Day care centers may be alternatives to institutional placement.

247. Pratt, Clara C. et al. "Burden and Coping Strategies of Caregivers to Alzheimer's Patients." *Family Relations*, v. 34, January 1985, pp. 27-33.

Taking care of Alzheimer's patients is extremely stressful. The investigators of this project examined the internal and external coping strategies used by the caregivers and the relationships of those strategies to the caregivers' subjective sense of burden.

248. Price, Joy Ann et al. "Elderly Persons' Perceptions and Knowledge of Alzheimer's Disease." *Psychological Reports*, v. 58, April 1986, pp. 419-424.

A study involving 148 elderly persons showed that the participants' knowledge of Alzheimer's disease was poor. Current media emphasis appears to have generated considerable fear of this disease among the elderly, but has resulted in very few effective education programs.

249. Rabins, Peter V. "Management of Dementia in the Family Context." *Psychosomatics*, v. 25, May 1984, pp. 369-375.

Alzheimer's disease has a dramatic impact on the families of its victims. Advice, reassurance, and other forms of support should be provided to these families through self-help groups, community agencies, and other types of professionals.

250. Reiffer, Burton V., Gary B. Cox, and Raymond J. Hanley. "Problems of Mentally Ill Elderly As Perceived By Patients, Families, and Clinicians." *Gerontologist*, v. 21, April 1981, pp. 165-170.

During the first year at a geriatric clinic for mentally ill members and their families, results showed that problems noted by a family were generally confirmed by a comprehensive clinical evaluation. However, the patients would underestimate or deny many of their own difficulties.

251. Schmidt, Gregory L. and Barbara Keyes. "Group Psychotherapy with Family Caregivers of Demented Patients." Gerontologist, v. 25, August 1985, pp. 347-350.

The need for support groups for Alzheimer's disease caregivers has been well documented over the past decade. The experiences of such a group are reported along with the dyamics of the transition from a support group to a therapy group.

252. Scott, Jean Pearson et al. "Families of Alzheimer's Victims: Family Support to the Caregivers." Journal of the American Geriatrics Society, v. 34, May 1986, pp. 348-354.

Family support is very helpful to those caring for Alzheimer's victims. The types of family assistance that this study showed to be most helpful to the primary caregiver were visits and having other persons stay with the patient. This enabled the primary caregiver to rest, get away for social activities, run errands, or even take a trip.

253. Sirovatka, Paul. "Heckler Announces Task Force on Alzheimer's Disease." Adamha News, v. 9, April 8, 1983, pp. 1-2.

The Secretary of Health and Human Services established a task force on Alzheimer's disease in 1983. The purpose of the task force was to coordinate research, provide a vehicle for translating that research into policy, develop programs, and improve the quality of life for older Americans.

254. U.S. Congress. House. Select Committee on Aging. Alzheimer's Disease: A Florida Perspective. Washington, DC: Government Printing Office, 1985. 79p. Superintendent of Documents Number Y4.Ag4/2:A19/4.

The text of a congressional hearing on the impact of Alzheimer's disease on its victims and their families. Resources need to be allocated to assist families in coping with the financial and emotional burden. Recommendations include day care programs, family support groups, and respite care days in nursing homes.

255. U.S. Congress. House. Select Committee on Aging. Alzheimer's Disease: Burdens and Problems for Victims and Their Families. Washington, DC: Government Printing Office, 1985. 58p. Superintendent of Documents Number Y4.Ag4/2:Al9/6.

A congressional hearing on one of the most serious problems facing senior citizens today: Alzheimer's disease. There is no viable long-term health care policy or method of repayment for the care of Alzheimer's patients.

256. U.S. Congress. House. Select Committee on Aging. Caring for America's Alzheimer's Victims. Washington, DC: Government Printing Office, 1985. 60p. Superintendent of Documents Number Y4.Ag4/2:Al9/5.

The text of testimony before Congress on what the federal government should do to provide care and assistance for Alzheimer's victims and their families.

257. U.S. Congress. House. Select Committee on Aging. Subcommittee on Health and Long-Term Care. Alzheimer's Disease: Joint Hearing. Washington, DC: Government Printing Office, 1984. 113p. Superintendent of Documents Number Y4.Ag4/2:Al9/3.

An appeal for more funds to research the causes and a cure for Alzheimer's disease and to try to provide some way for families to receive care assistance.

258. U.S. Congress. House. Select Committee on Aging. Subcommittee on Health and Long-Term Care. Alzheimer's Disease: Pennsylvania Perspective. Washington, DC: Government Printing Office, 1986. 58p. Superintendent of Documents Number Y4.Ag4/2:Al9/7.

It is important for policymakers to have a clear understanding of Alzheimer's disease and its implications for health and aging policy at all levels. Testimony is presented from an attorney who devotes a large portion of his practice to counseling families of Alzheimer's patients on patient and family rights and responsibilities.

259. U.S. Congress. House. Select Committee on Aging. Subcommittee on Health and Long-Term Care. <u>Long-Term Care: Need for a National Policy</u>. Washington, DC: Government Printing Office, 1984. 115p. Superintendent of Documents Number Y4.Ag4/2:C18/corr.

    The United States has no long-term health care policy. Nowhere in our society are families left so unassisted as they are in meeting the financial and emotional burden of caring for an Alzheimer's patient.

260. U.S. Congress. Senate. Special Committee on Aging. <u>Endless Night, Endless Mourning: Living with Alzheimer's</u>. Washington, DC: Government Printing Office, 1983. 72p. Superintendent of Documents Number Y4.Ag4:S.hrg.98-410.

    The text of a hearing to investigate the medical and social service needs of Alzheimer's patients and families.

261. Wasow, Mona. "Support Groups for Family Caregivers of Patients with Alzheimer's Disease." <u>Social Work</u>, v. 31, March/April 1986, pp. 93-97.

    Describes the experiences of a social worker who has worked with a support group for family caregivers of patients with Alzheimer's disease. A model of an ideal support group program is provided.

262. Williams-Schroeder, Mary L. "Meeting the Needs of the Alzheimer's Caregiver." <u>Physical and Occupational Therapy in Geriatrics</u>, v. 3, Summer 1984, pp. 33-38.

    The educational, emotional, physical, social, and professional needs of those who care for Alzheimer's victims are very great. Means must be worked out for dealing with the stress which this disorder creates among the staff and families caring for Alzheimer's patients.

263. Zarit, Steven H., Nancy K. Orr, and Judy M. Zarit. <u>The Hidden Victims of Alzheimer's Disease: Families Under Stress</u>. New York, New York University Press, 1985. 218p. ISBN 0-8147-9662-1.

    The families who act as caretakers are the hidden victims of Alzheimer's disease. They must receive support through groups, counseling, and additional support services and research.

264. Zarit, Steven H., Nancy K. Orr, and Judy M. Zarit. <u>Working with Families of Dementia Victims: A Treatment Manual.</u> Washington, DC: Government Printing Office, 1983. 150p. Superintendent of Documents Number HE23.3008:A19/v.4.

A handbook for both professionals and the families of Alzheimer's victims and a source to help understand senile dementia. Causes, symptoms, guidelines for assessment and treatment, and needed policy changes are covered.

265. Zarit, Steven H., Karen E. Reever, and Julie Bach-Peterson. "Relatives of the Impaired Elderly: Correlates of Feeling of Burden." <u>Gerontologist</u>, v. 20, December 1980, pp. 649-655.

The importance of providing support to caregivers is emphasized in this study of primary caregivers of senile dementia patients living at home. Feelings of burden were lessened when frequent visits were paid by other relatives.

266. Zinsser, John. "Alzheimer's a Funding Priority." <u>50 Plus</u>, v. 24, December 1984, pp. 12-13.

The $1.26 billion Older Americans Act earmarked $36 million for five Alzheimer's biomedical research centers. The act also makes provisions for support for family caregivers in the form of transportation services, adult day care, and tax credits for certain users of day care facilities.

Author Index

Name: Abstract Number.

Adamo, J.: 208.
Almind, G.: 94.
Anderton, B.: 135.
Arehart-Freichel, J.: 137, 138.
Aronson, M.: 229, 230.
Arp, J.: 195.
Arrington, C.: 96.
Atkins, M. H.: 209.
Bach-Peterson, J.: 265.
Ball, M. J.: 139.
Barlow, A. R.: 210.
Barnes, R. F.: 231.
Barry, P. P.: 43.
Becker, J.: 245.
Benson, D. F.: 192.
Berger, E. Y.: 97.
Berman, S.: 232.
Besson, J. A. O.: 140.
Black, B. C.: 7.
Blass, J. P.: 3.
Bloom, F.: 141.
Bock, F. A.: 244.
Brandt, A.: 211.
Breitner, J. C. S.: 85.
Brody, E. M.: 190.
Brown, D. S.: 98.
Butler, R. N.: 142.
Buys, D.: 99.
Bylinsky, G.: 143.
Carey, J.: 47.
Carnes, M.: 79.
Charles, L.: 4.
Check, W.: 144.
Clark, M.: 5, 145, 146.
Cohen, D.: 101, 102, 154.
Cohen, G. D.: 198.
Coppel, D. B.: 245.
Corkin, S.: 149.
Courtice, K.: 122.
Cox, G. B.: 250.
Cox, K. G.: 103.
Crane, N.: 195.
Crook, T. H.: 191.
Crossman, L.: 234.

Cummings, J. L.: 80, 192.
Cutler, N. R.: 104.
Cybyk, M. E.: 235.
Dalessio, D. J.: 193.
David, I.: 6.
David, L.: 6.
Demak, R.: 81.
Dickstein, E. S.: 82.
Dilka, C.: 236.
Doubleday, O. A.: 212.
Dougherty, J. H.: 202.
Duara, R.: 7.
Edwards, D. D.: 150.
Edwards, D. E.: 8.
Edwards, H.: 83.
Eide, M.: 151.
Eisdorfer, C.: 101.
Emr, M.: 9, 152, 153, 180.
English, D.: 154.
Feil, N.: 194.
Fein, E.: 11.
Finch, C. E.: 156.
Fine, A.: 157.
Finlayson, A.: 12.
Finlinson, R.: 84.
Finn, R.: 13.
Fischman, J.: 14, 158.
Folkenberg, J.: 105, 160.
Folstein, M. F.: 85.
Footer, M.: 15.
Forsythe, J.: 161.
Francis, P. T.: 162.
Frank, J.: 16.
Freedman, G. A.: 17.
French, L. R.: 55.
Friedland, R. P.: 87.
Ghazarbekian, B.: 213.
Glaze, B.: 214.
Glenner, G. G.: 163.
Glosser, G.: 237.
Goldberg, R. T.: 106.
Golden, R. R.: 88.
Goldsmith, M. F.: 18, 107, 164.
Goodman, G.: 108.
Gosnell, M.: 145.
Grady, D.: 56.
Gray, A.: 57.
Greene, J. A.: 109, 195.
Gurland, B. J.: 88.

Gwyther, L. P.: 110.
Hamilton, H. L.: 21.
Hanley, R. J.: 250.
Harrington-Hughes, K.: 21.
Haugen, P. K.: 111.
Hayter, J.: 238.
Hecht, A.: 22.
Heckler, M. M.: 23.
Hemshorn, A.: 215.
Herbert, W.: 165, 196.
Herz, L. R.: 132.
Hinton, D. R.: 166.
Hirschfeld, M.: 239.
Hoeft, T. M.: 243.
Holland, G. B.: 216.
Hollister, A.: 217.
Hubbard, L.: 24.
Hutton, J. T.: 167.
Jarvis, J.: 218.
Jenike, M. A.: 58.
Johnson, J.: 112.
Kahan, J.: 240.
Katzman, R.: 168.
Kelly, W. E.: 169.
Kenny, A. D.: 167.
Kent, S.: 59.
Keyes, B.: 251.
Khachaturian, Z. S.: 170.
Klumph, L. F.: 25.
Kolata, G.: 171.
Kromm, D.: 113.
Kromm, Y. H. N.: 113.
Kvale, J. N.: 26.
LaBarge, E.: 241.
Lauter, H.: 27.
Lazarus, L. W.: 242.
Lerner, M. R.: 219.
Levy, R.: 172.
Lindeman, D. A.: 28.
Lunzer, F.: 29.
MacDonald, D. I.: 60.
Mace, N. L.: 114, 197.
Mahendra, B.: 61.
Makohon, R.: 117.
Marois, M.: 53.
Martin, A.: 173.
Martinson, I. M.: 30.
Matteson, M. A.: 110.
Mayeux, R.: 31.

McAuliffe, S.: 174.
McGowan, A.: 32.
Mercer, M.: 33.
Middleton, L.: 115.
Miller, J. A.: 175.
Miller, N. E.: 191, 198.
Miot, C.: 199.
Mobily, K. E.: 243.
Mohs, R. C.: 176.
Montgomery, R,: 116.
Mortimer, J. A.: 62.
Narang, P. K.: 104.
Nee, L.: 64.
Newell, J.: 177.
Ninos, M.: 117.
Nolen, W. A.: 66.
Oliver, R.: 244.
Orr, N. K.: 263, 264.
Pagel, M. D.: 245.
Palmer, M. H.: 119.
Panella, J. J.: 246.
Pardes, H.: 178.
Parker, J. C.: 201.
Paschke, M. J.: 120.
Peppard, N. R.: 121.
Powell, L. S.: 35, 122.
Powers, L. B.: 202.
Pratt, C. C.: 247.
Pressler, L.: 220.
Price, D. L.: 89.
Price, J. A.: 248.
Rabins, P. V.: 114, 123, 249.
Racz, T. M.: 151.
Rappaport, M. B.: 232.
Reever, K. E.: 207, 265.
Reiffer, B. V.: 250.
Reisberg, B.: 67, 90, 124, 179.
Ricci, M.: 125.
Richards, L. D.: 36.
Ringland, E.: 126.
Roach, M.: 221-223.
Rosen, W. G.: 31.
Rosenfeld, I.: 69.
Rovner, J.: 37.
Sabin, T. D.: 91.
Safford, F.: 127.
Sands, D.: 128.
Santini, R.: 224.
Sargent, M.: 38, 39.

Schafer, S. C.: 129.
Schmidt, G. L.: 251.
Schneider, E. L.: 180.
Schuman, L. M.: 62.
Schwab, M.: 130.
Scileppi, K. P.: 181.
Scott, J. P.: 252.
Seymour, C.: 225.
Shodell, M.: 41.
Shore, D.: 183.
Shuttleworth, E. C.: 92.
Silberner, J.: 184.
Sirovatka, P.: 253.
Steel, K.: 43.
Stern, M. B.: 203.
Storandt, M.: 70.
Suzuki, T.: 128.
Teresi, J. A.: 88.
Terry, R. D.: 71.
Thomas, L.: 44.
Tisdale, S.: 205.
Tolliver, L. M.: 45.
Toseland, R. W.: 46.
Trafford, A.: 47.
Trubo, R.: 72.
Truesdell, M. L.: 4.
Volicer, L.: 132.
Wallis, C.: 52.
Wasow, M.: 261.
Wertheimer, J.: 53.
Wexler, D.: 237.
Whall, A.: 93.
Wheater, R. H.: 187.
White, J. A.: 188.
Williams-Schroeder, M. L.: 262.
Wisniewski, K. E.: 206.
Witherspoon, D.: 146.
Wood, E. L.: 4.
Woodward, J.: 226.
Wooll, A. C.: 227.
Wurtman, R.: 76.
Wyngaarden, J. B.: 77.
Yatzkan, E. S.: 229.
Zachary, R. A.: 133.
Zarit, J. M.: 207, 263, 264.
Zarit, S. H.: 207, 263-265.
Zinsser, J.: 266.

LIBRARY USE ONLY
DOES NOT CIRCULATE